PROFESSIONAL SERVICES FOR MEN:
HAIRCOLORING AND HAIR RESTORATION

THOMSON

DELMAR LEARNING

Australia   Canada   Mexico   Singapore   Spain   United Kingdom   United States

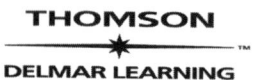

Milady's Professional Services for Men: Haircoloring and Hair Restoration

President, Milady:
Dawn Gerrain

Director of Learning Solutions:
Sherry Dickinson

Acquisitions Editor:
Brad Hanson

Product Manager:
Erik Herman

Editorial Assistant:
Jessica Burns

Director of Content and Media Productions:
Wendy A. Troeger

Content Project Manager:
Nina Tucciarelli

Associate Content Project Manager:
Angela Iula

Composition:
Carlisle Publishing Services

Director of Marketing:
Wendy Mapstone

Marketing Channel Manager:
Sandra Bruce

Marketing Coordinator:
Nicole Riggi

Cover Design:
Essence of Seven

Library of Congress Cataloging-in-Publication Data:
Milady's professional services for men : haircoloring and hair restoration.
    p. cm. — (Professional services for men)
Includes index.
ISBN-10: 1-4180-5090-3
ISBN-13: 978-1-4018-8169-6
1. Barbering. 2. Hair—Dyeing and bleaching. 3. Wigs. I. Milady Publishing Company. II. Series.
TT957.M55155 2007
646.7'24—dc22

                          2006016613

NOTICE TO THE READER

Publisher does not warrant or guarantee any of the products described herein or perform any independent analysis in connection with any of the product information contained herein. Publisher does not assume, and expressly disclaims, any obligation to obtain and include information other than that provided to it by the manufacturer.

The reader is expressly warned to consider and adopt all safety precautions that might be indicated by the activities herein and to avoid all potential hazards. By following the instructions contained herein, the reader willingly assumes all risks in connection with such instructions.

The publisher makes no representation or warranties of any kind, including but not limited to the warranties of fitness for particular purpose or merchantabiity, nor are any such representations implied with respect to the material set forth herein, and the publisher takes no responsibility with respect to such material. The publisher shall not be liable for any special, consequential, or exemplary damages resulting, in whole or part, from the readers' use of, or reliance upon, this material.

TABLE OF CONTENTS

2   HAIRCOLORING AND LIGHTENING / 33

PREFACE

A resurgence of barbers, barbershops, and barbering is taking place nationwide as the male consumer once again seeks the ambience and services of a real barbershop. To meet the growing needs and demands of their male clientele, many shops are finding they must offer a full range of professional hair and skin care services for men—it is no longer enough to offer just a good cut. Have you found yourself in this position? Are you an experienced barber who needs to learn more about male skin care and facial hair design? Are you interested in managing your own shop? Do you know all there is to know about cutting and styling but are interested in exploring haircoloring or hair restoration? Do you want to add men's services to your salon or day spa and need information specific to caring for male clientele? Or, are you new to the profession and want to learn about the fundamentals of cutting and styling, or seek a barbering position? Whatever the case may be, the *Professional Services for Men* series is for you.

Thomson Delmar Learning has created a series of concise, informative books designed to help licensed barbers and stylists develop the skills necessary to meet the growing needs of their male clientele. The four books in the series are:

Professional Services for Men: Facial Massage, Shaving and Hair Design

Professional Services for Men: Haircoloring and Hair Restoration

Professional Services for Men: Haircutting and Styling

Professional Services for Men: Career Management for Barbers

Each book presents the need-to-know information in an easy to understand format. Utilizing numerous full-color images and drawings, straightforward language, and and helpful features such as "Tech Terms," "FYI," "Caution," and "Focus On," for added learning enrichment in your profession. To enhance your learning, the first three books take you step-by-step through the fundamental techniques of hair and skin care for men while emphasizing client comfort and safety. The last book in the *Professional Services for Men* series moves away from the technical aspects of providing men's services and looks toward the career management side of the profession.

In this, the second book in the series, we explore the exciting areas of hair restoration and hair coloring. As noted, more and more men are taking an interest in their appearance and, as a result, are seeking these image-enhancing services. In *Section 1, Hair Restoration,* you will find an overview of the various hair restoration options available. Though the emphasis in this section is on *nonsurgical* hair replacement options, such as *hairpieces* and *wigs,* you will also find information on the *surgical, pharmaceutical,* and *hair weave* options available. In addition, you will find suggestions for selling and marketing nonsurgical hair replacement services to your clients. Finally, to assist you in providing those services, you will find detailed information on how to *mea-*

sure, clean, apply, cut, style, color, permanent wave, and *care for* a hairpiece or wig. This information will enable you to keep your clients' nonsurgical hair replacements looking and feeling good.

In *Section 2,* you will learn the fundamentals about haircoloring and lightening, including information about the *structure of hair, color theory, haircoloring products,* and *haircolor terminology.* You will also learn how to perform key tasks such as the *haircoloring consultation* and the *patch, strand,* and *metallic salts and coating dyes tests.* In addition, you will learn the basics about *coloring gray hair, reconditioning damaged hair, removing coatings from hair,* and *coloring mustaches and beards.* You will also find step-by-step procedures for *applying a temporary color rinse, semipermanent color,* or *single-process color; lightening virgin hair; applying toners and lighteners;* and *performing single-process color retouches.* Finally, you will find a summary of the *safety precautions* that must be taken to ensure a successful and safe haircoloring or lightening service.

So, if you are ready to learn the ins and outs of hair restoration and hair coloring, turn the page and let the journey begin!

A very special thank you to the following individuals for their contributions and assistance with the Professional Men's Services series:

Maura T. Scali-Sheahan, Master Barber and Educator
Cory Cole, Master Barber
Vinny Federico, Master Barber
Laura Downs, Barber
Greg Zorian, Jr., Master Barber
Greg Zorian, III, Master Barber
Helen Wos, Instructor/Barber
Lorilee Bird, Student Barber
Mark Blue, Student Barber
Christopher Morris, Student Barber
Kristen Santa Lucia, Student Barber

Andis, William Marvy Company, Wahl, and 44/20 for use of their product photographs.

Gregory's Barbershop, Clifton Park, NY for use of their location.

Morris Flamingo, Inc. for use of the Campbell Lather King.

Photography Credits:

Section 1: Section Opener photo, Figures 1a–10, 12–20, Paul Castle Photography
Section 2: Section Opener photo, Figures 35–40, 43–67, Paul Castle Photography
Figures 21, 68, 69, provided by Milady

PROFESSIONAL SERVICES FOR MEN:
HAIRCOLORING AND HAIR RESTORATION

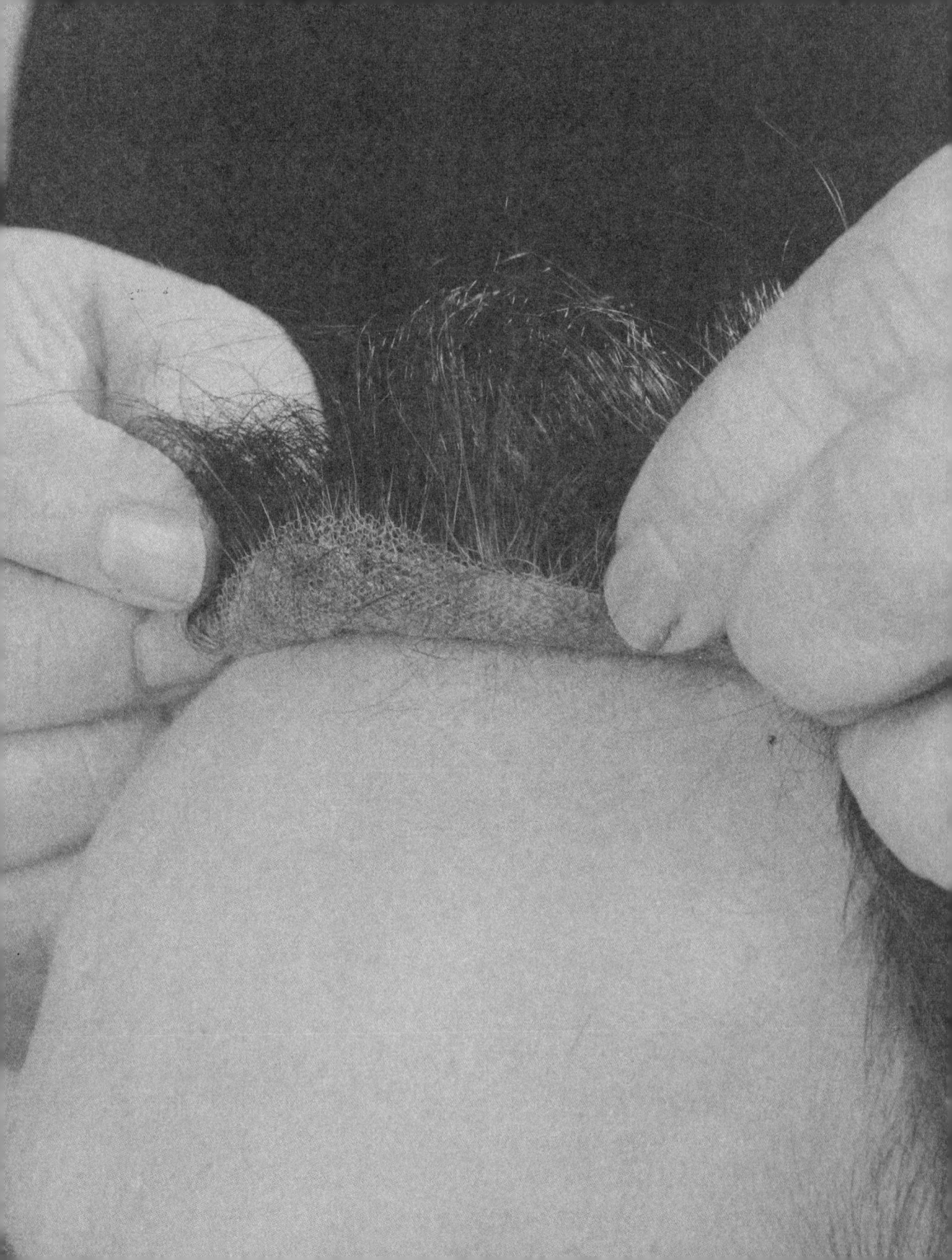

MEN'S NONSURGICAL HAIR REPLACEMENTS

1

SECTION TOPICS

HAIRPIECE QUALITY

MEASURING FOR THE HAIRPIECE

CLEANING AND STYLING HAIRPIECES

ALTERNATIVE HAIR RESTORATION TECHNIQUES

From early Assyrian, Egyptian, and Roman times, hairpieces and wigs have been worn in an attempt to cover balding pates, as a part of ceremonial ritual or in conformance with the prevailing fashion. False beards and mustaches, dreadlocks, full-bottom wigs, partial wigs, periwigs, side rolls, bobbed wigs, clubs, and queues have all played a role in this history, from ancient times to the present. During the 18th century, the word *toupee* was used to describe the front section of hair known as the foretop. This section of hair was grown long enough to cover the front part of the wig, which was placed farther back on the head in order to blend the natural hair with the artificial wig hair. Over time, the foretop was combed higher and extended back toward the crown until it became one long tail of hair. Today, the term *toupee* has come to mean a small, nonsurgical hair replacement, or hairpiece, that is used to cover the top or crown of the head. These terms will be used interchangeably throughout Section 1.

For centuries, barbers were involved with the making and styling of hairpieces. Today, the care and fitting of men's hairpieces in the barbershop continues the traditions established so long ago. Although not all barbers choose to specialize in nonsurgical hair replacement services, the professional who can design, fit, and custom-cut a hairpiece can open the door to increased clientele and financial gain.

Men wear hairpieces for a variety of personal reasons that originate from the desire to cover thinning or balding areas of the head. Studies have shown that hair loss definitely has an emotional impact; although the medical community does not recognize this as a medical condition, many individuals with a hair loss condition feel anguish that is real and often overlooked. One study that investigated the perceptions of bald and balding men compared to men who had hair revealed that bald men were perceived as being less physically attractive (by both sexes), less assertive, less successful, less personally likeable, and older looking. Though these actual characteristics might not have been true, such perceptions can influence the emotions and thoughts of a man who is losing his hair.

According to the studies, the perceptions that bald men have of themselves, as compared to those with moderate hair loss, revealed that they experience more negative and emotional effects, are more preoccupied with their baldness, and make some effort to conceal or compensate for their hair loss. Given these self-perceptions, it is understandable why men might choose the hair restoration options available to them (Figures 1a and 1b).

Hair restoration techniques range from topical applications of drugs such as minoxidil to toupees to surgical hair transplantation and scalp reduction. This section focuses primarily on men's hairpieces, with a brief discussion of other alternatives available to men with hair loss conditions.

■ TECH TERM

Topical refers to the application of a preparation directly to the skin, rather than through ingestion.

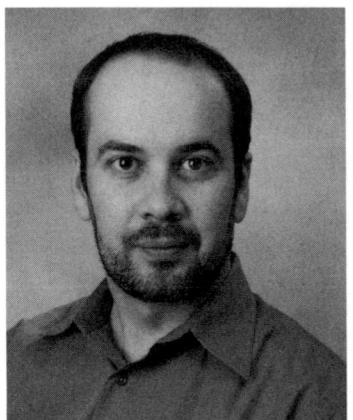

FIGURE 1A │ Before nonsurgical hair replacement.

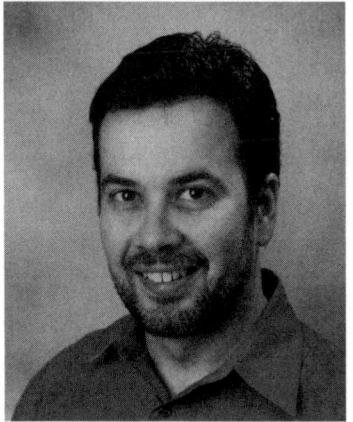

FIGURE 1B │ After nonsurgical hair replacement.

■ | HAIRPIECE QUALITY

The quality of a hairpiece varies with the kind of hair used in its manufacture and the way in which it is constructed. The barber is often the one to measure, fit, cut, and style the hairpiece once it has been received from the supplier.

Human Hair

Human hair is usually the most desirable choice for a quality hairpiece, although synthetic fibers, such as Kanekalon, effectively simulate the look and touch of human hair. The advantages of human hair include a more natural look and texture, durability, and the ability to tolerate chemical process such as permanent waving or hair coloring. Some of the disadvantages associated with a human hair hairpiece is that it will react to climate changes and fade with exposure to light, requires styling maintenance, and can become damaged just as natural hair can. Human hair hairpieces are usually cleaned with a dry-cleaning solvent. Always follow the manufacturer's directions.

The most expensive hairpieces are made from human hair, and often originate from Europe or Asia. Most hair from India tends to have a natural wave pattern whereas Asian hair is usually straight. Human hair blends are also available that use animal hair in the construction of the hairpiece. Yet a third option is to use the client's own hair from thick-growth areas and then have it made into a hairpiece by one of the many hair clubs specializing in that technique.

Most of the human hair used in hairpieces is imported and must be prepared for use. The process usually includes chemical cleaning with an acid solution, sorting, and root-turning, which means that all the hair is sewn into the base with the hair cuticle of the strands flowing in the same direction.

Synthetic Hair

Synthetic hair is used primarily in the production of full wigs, rather than toupees. It is challenging to make synthetic hair that matches the texture of human hair, which makes it difficult to blend the piece with the client's natural hair. Synthetic fibers also possess a high gloss that makes them more noticeable, and when blended with human or animal hair, they tend to mat and tangle easily. Overall, synthetic hairpieces can usually be cleaned with water and shampoo, are less costly than human hair, and do not oxidize or lose the style.

Mixed Hair

Mixed-hair products, such as human hair blended with animal hair, are often used in the manufacture of theatrical or fashion wigs. Horse and yak hair, as well as angora and sheep's wool, are the types of materials used in the manufacture of hairpieces. Angora has a finer texture than yak and is often used at the front hairline to create a soft and more natural look.

For the barber who is interested in servicing and supplying hairpieces to clients, it is advisable to study this area of the industry in detail. There will be decisions to make about manufacturers, supplies, products, and equipment; these can be made intelligently only with a thorough understanding of the business.

In selecting a hairpiece manufacturer to work with there are many important questions to ask. The following is a representative sample of some questions that will require answers before a manufacturer can be selected to provide hairpiece goods to the barbershop.

- What hair materials are used in the construction of the hairpiece: human, synthetic, or mixed?
- Is the hair in a virgin state or have chemical treatments been applied? If so, what?

- ◘ If the hair is human hair, is it graded in terms of strength, elasticity, and porosity?

- ◘ Has the hairpiece been root-turned?

- ◘ What is the life expectancy of the hairpiece?

- ◘ Will the manufacturer match the client's natural hair color?

Bases and Construction

Hairpieces are available with hard, soft, mesh, net, polyurethane, or combination bases. Soft-base hairpieces usually have a base material of silk gauze, nylon mesh, or plastic mesh. The better hairpieces will be made with a doubled base material for increased strength and a more exact fit. Double-knotted hair in the hairpiece ensures that the hair remains intact through use and cleaning. Conversely, single-knot hairpieces may come untied during the cleaning process due to alcohol-based solvents, which can weaken the hair. Plastic or nylon-mesh bases resist shrinkage and wrinkling when cleaned in water-based solutions or shampoos.

New construction techniques with more natural-looking materials are constantly evolving in the manufacture of hairpieces. Some of the standard types of construction are as follows:

- ◘ *Wefted* hairpieces are usually machine-made. Wefts are strips of material or thread to which the hair is sewn. Most wefts are spaced for balance and proper hair distribution when sewn onto a mesh cap.

- ◘ Handmade, *hand-tied* hairpieces are costly because each hair strand is sewn in individually. These pieces are usually ventilated and comfortable to wear.

- ◘ *Lace-front* hairpieces consist of a silk gauze foundation with a lace-edged front; they are suitable for pompadour or parted hairstyles that are combed away from the face.

- *Hard-base* hairpieces are made of plastics and resins into which the hair is positioned before the material hardens. The hair is rooted in a specific design and direction, thus this style of hairpiece is less flexible than some other types.

- *Soft-base* hairpiece materials usually consist of silk gauze, nylon mesh, or plastic mesh.

Stock and Custom Hairpieces

Hairpieces are available from manufacturers and distributors in stock sizes and colors, which allows the barber to maintain an inventory of these products. Stock hairpieces can be used as samples to show prospective nonsurgical hair replacement clients how a toupee may look, or may be customized by the barber to fit the client.

Custom hairpieces are obviously more tailored to each client's head shape and hair restoration needs because the barber creates a pattern and color matching for the supplier to use as a guide in the production of the hairpiece.

A pattern or contour analysis should be done prior to fitting any hairpiece. This analysis will help to determine whether the client has the option of purchasing a stock product or requires a custom-made hairpiece.

Supplies for Hairpiece Services

Most barbershops will already have many of the implements and supplies required for hairpiece services (Figure 2). The items that may not be standard can be obtained from a barber or hairpiece supply company. Be guided by the following checklist when purchasing hairpiece service supplies:

- acetone or remover solvent

- alcohol

- blow-dryer

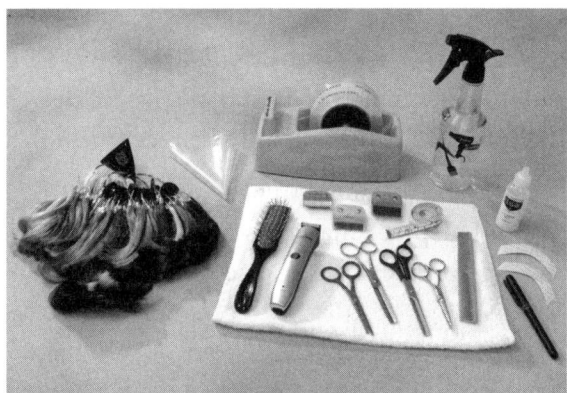

FIGURE 2 | Supplies for hairpiece services.

- client record cards
- clippers
- comb
- double-sided adhesive tape
- envelopes
- grease pencil
- hair net
- haircutting shears
- measuring tape
- plastic wrap
- razor
- scissors (for cutting pattern)
- small brush
- spirit gum
- styling block
- thinning shears
- T-pins
- transparent tape
- wig cleaner

■ | MEASURING FOR THE HAIRPIECE

Once the client consultation has been performed and an understanding has been reached about the type of non-surgical hair replacement to be purchased, a preliminary haircut should be performed.

To achieve a natural look, the client's hair should be allowed to grow fairly long to make it easier to blend it with that of the hairpiece. When performing the preliminary cut, the hair should be lightly trimmed, leaving a long neckline and length close to the ears at the sides. Make sure to trim the front section as well (Figure 3). After the preliminary cut is finished, the longest cuttings are gathered and put into an envelope for use as a texture and color guide for the manufacturer.

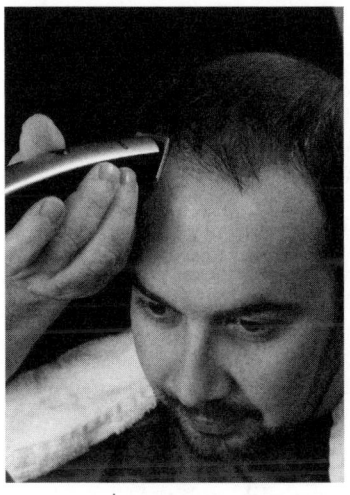

FIGURE 3 | Trim the front section.

The sizes of men's hairpieces are commonly measured in inches. For example, a 6-by-4-inch piece would be 6 inches long from front to back, and 4 inches wide. In the manufacturer's code, the larger number refers to the length unless otherwise indicated. Tape measurements alone can be used for ordering stock hairpieces. Custom pieces, however, require a pattern of the client's head form in the area of hair loss.

▷ procedure no. 1

Hairpiece Pattern Making

Tape Measurement

For a front hairline to look natural, it should not be too low on the forehead. The original and natural hairline should be followed as closely as possible. The following procedure is a standard method of measuring for a hairpiece.

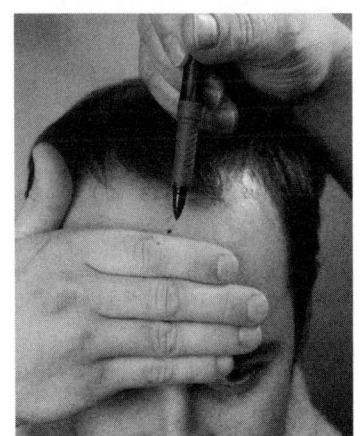

FIGURE 4 | Mark the center where the hairpiece will begin.

1   Place four fingers above the eyebrow with the last finger resting on the bridge of the nose. Make a dot with a grease pencil on the forehead directly in line with the center of the nose to indicate where the hairpiece is to begin (Figure 4).

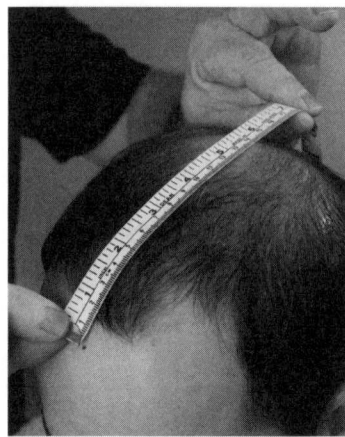

FIGURE 5 | Measure from the dot to the back section.

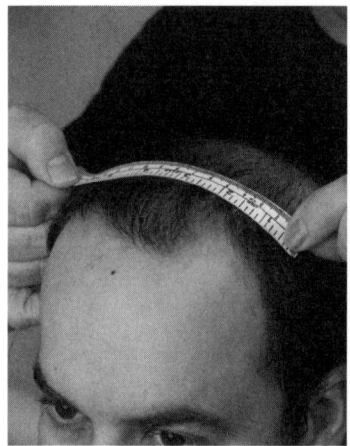

FIGURE 6 | Measure across the top.

2 Place the tape measure on the dot. Measure the length to where the back hair begins and mark the tape measure. Be sure to measure back to where substantial growth begins and disregard sparse hair between the forehead and bald crown areas (Figure 5).

3 The next measurement is across the top, directly over the sideburn. This is the place where the front hairline of the hairpiece blends in with the client's own hair at the sides of the head. Measure across the crown area if it is noticeably different from the front width (Figure 6). These measurements can be used to order a stock hairpiece.

Pattern Measurements

To create a pattern for a custom hairpiece, assemble the measuring tape, plastic wrap, 12 strips of 3/4-inch transparent tape (preferably the dull-finish type for easy writing), and a grease pencil.

1 Place approximately 2 feet of plastic wrap on top of the client's head and twist the sides until they conform to the contour of the head.

2 Place three fingers above the eyebrows and make a dot on the pattern to indicate the new hairline. Place additional dots as follows:
   a. two dots on each side where the front hairline is to meet the client's own hairline
   b. two dots in back of the head on each side of the balding spot
   c. one dot at the center back edge of the bald spot to determine the length of the area to be covered

3 Connect the dots with a pencil to outline the balding area (Figure 7). Ignore minor irregularities and sparse areas.

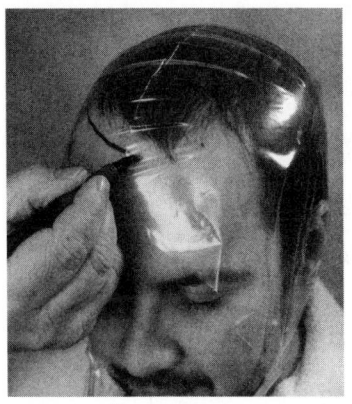

FIGURE 7 | Apply plastic wrap and connect the dots.

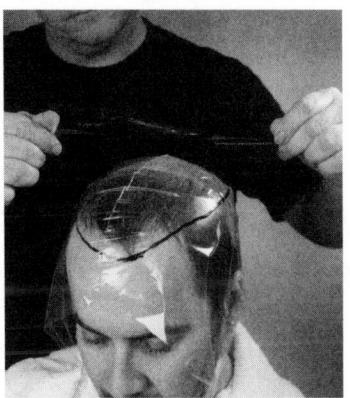

FIGURE 8 | Place tape across the bald area to stiffen the pattern.

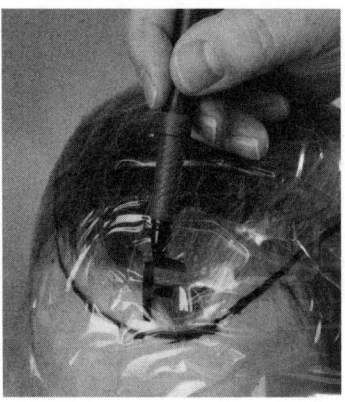

FIGURE 9 | Mark the front (F) and back (B) on the pattern.

4 While the client holds the plastic wrap, place each precut strip of tape across the bald area to stiffen the pattern and hold its shape (Figure 8).

5 Mark the front part of the pattern F and the back B, as in Figure 9. Then remove and cut around the edge with scissors. After cutting the outline, replace the pattern over the balding area (Figure 10). Make sure the bald area is covered exactly. Although it is better to have a foundation that is slightly smaller than one that is too large, accuracy is very important.

6 Attach samples of the client's hair to the pattern or client card for color matching by the manufacturer.

7 Create a client record card (Figure 11), which can also serve as an information sheet when ordering stock and custom hairpieces. Send the measurements and/or pattern to the manufacturer with instructions covering the information in Figure 11.

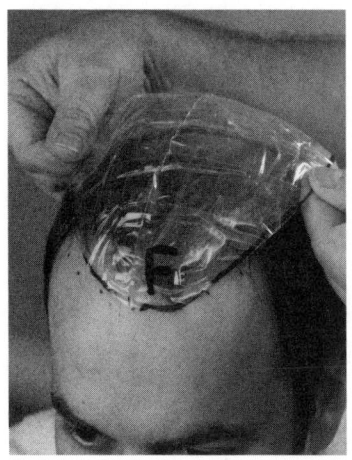

FIGURE 10 | Check fit and size of pattern.

1. Hairpiece without lace front (Figure 16-11)

   a) Without side part   ☐

   b) With left side part   ☐

   c) With right side part   ☐

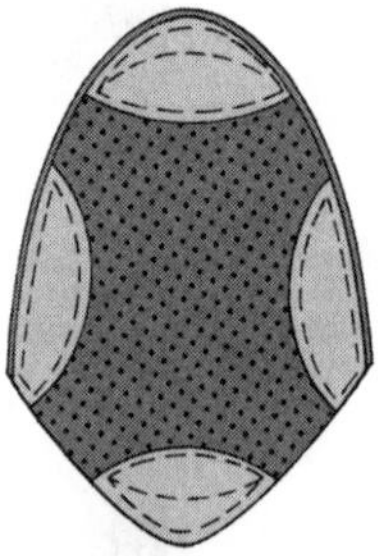

2. Hairpiece with lace front (Figure 16-12)

   a) With side part   ☐

   b) With left side part   ☐

   c) With right side part   ☐

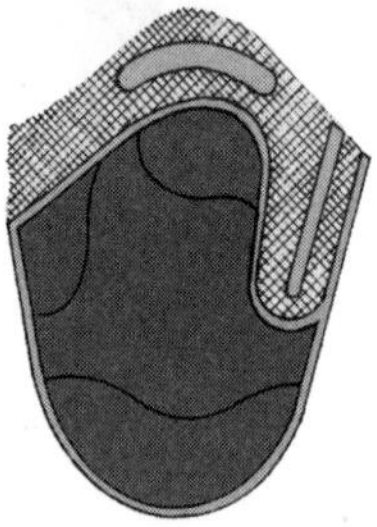

3. Hair color variations:

a) Front:	Natural	☐	Percentage of gray	☐
	Streaked	☐	Front and top lighter	☐
b) Temples:	Natural	☐	Percentage of gray	☐
c) Back:	Natural	☐	Percentage of gray	☐

4. Complexion:

   a)   Ruddy: ☐

   b)   Dark: ☐

   c)   Light: ☐

5. Details:

   a)   Partials ☐   Patches ☐   Fill-ins ☐

6. Photograph (may or may not be required by manufacturer).

FIGURE 11 | Client record card.

▷ procedure no. 2

Applying a Non-Lace, Front Hairpiece

1 Before adjusting a hairpiece to the scalp, trim the front hairline and clean the entire bald area with a piece of cotton dampened with rubbing alcohol, or soap and water, then dry thoroughly.

2 Apply two-sided tape in a V-shape on the front reinforced area of the foundation (Figure 12). This tape holds the hairpiece close to the scalp. Place additional pieces of tape on the reinforced parts of the foundation at the sides and back of the hairpiece.

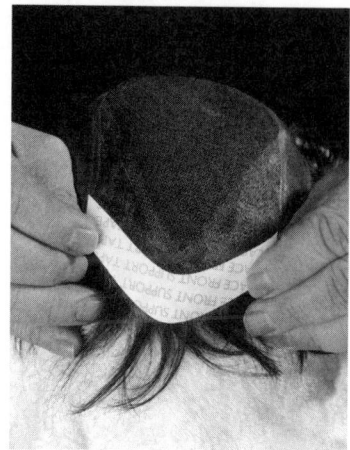

FIGURE 12 │ Apply two-sided tape in V-shape.

3 Place three fingers above the eyebrow to locate the hairline. Position the hairpiece at the hairline using the center of the nose as a guide. When the hairpiece is in the proper position, press down firmly on the various tape areas (Figure 13).

Cutting, Tapering, and Blending the Hairpiece

- *Back and sides.* When the hair is combed into the desired position, use a razor or shears to taper and blend the hair smoothly at the back of the head. Then taper and blend the sides. The tapering should be done gradually so that the blending with the client's natural hair will be undetectable.

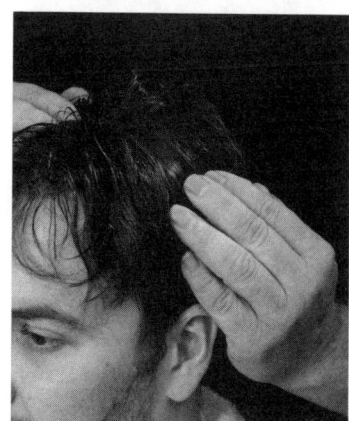

FIGURE 13 │ Attach the hairpiece, press down firmly on taped areas.

- *Top section.* Depending on the density of the hairpiece, the fingers-and-shear method may be used to cut in the top section. Comb the hair up, bring it slightly forward, and cut. Repeat this operation as needed to blend using shears or thinning shears.

- *Blend crest with front.* Use the razor to blend the hairpiece with the natural side hair in the crest area. Cut a small

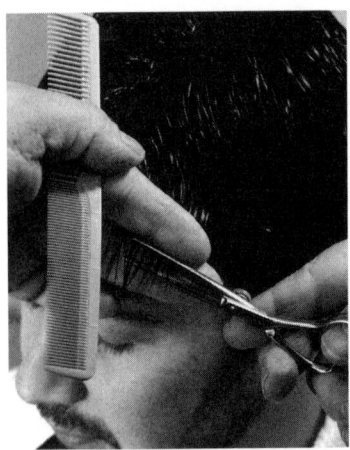

FIGURE 14 | Trim front sections.

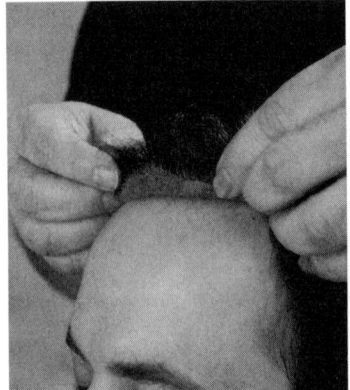

FIGURE 15 | Removing a hairpiece.

amount of front hair short to soften the joining of the hairpiece with the client's hair (Figure 14).

◻ *Thick front hairline.* If the front hairline appears heavy, use a razor for thinning. Be sure to make very narrow partings in order to form a natural-looking front hairline. To thin underneath hair, comb the hair forward and thin it with a razor. When combed back, the hair should lie flat.

NOTE: *For detailed information on haircutting techniques, including razor cutting, see* Professional Services for Men: Haircutting and Styling.

◻ *Removing a hairpiece.* Reach up under the hairpiece with the fingertips at the front section and detach the tape from the scalp (Figure 15). Make sure the tape stays on the foundation so that it can be reactivated with spirit gum.

▷ procedure no. 3

Applying a Lace-Front Hairpiece

A hairpiece with a lace front is recommended when the hair is worn in an off-the-face style. It is scarcely visible from the front view and provides the required lightness for a natural-looking hairstyle.

1   Clean the bald area with rubbing alcohol or with soap and water.

2   Remove hair on the scalp where the tape or lace is to be attached (Figure 16).

3   Attach strips of tape (two-sided) to reinforced parts of the foundation, usually near the front, on the sides, and the back part of the hairpiece. Note that

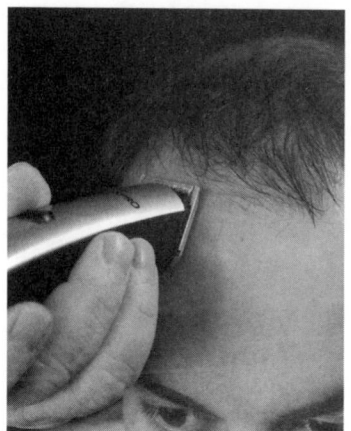

FIGURE 16 | Remove hair on scalp where the hairpiece will attach.

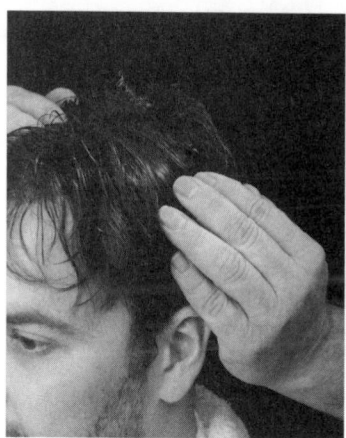

FIGURE 17 | Adjust the hairpiece.

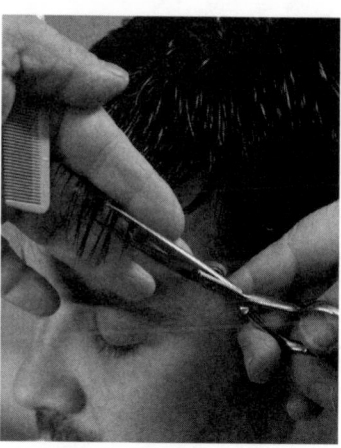

FIGURE 18 | Cut, taper, and blend the hairpiece with the client's natural hair.

reinforced areas vary with the design of the foundation and the manufacturer's specifications. Never apply tape directly to the lace.

4   Adjust the hairpiece to the desired position using the three-finger method. Press it down into place (Figure 17).

5   Cut, taper, and blend the front-lace hairpiece to match smoothly with the client's own hair (Figure 18).

6   Trim the lace to within 1/4 of an inch of the hairline, or right down to the contour of the hairline, according to the client's preference.

NOTE: The decision to trim or not to trim should be left until the hairpiece has been worn for a while. In the beginning, leave a small, 1/4-inch margin.

Removing a lace-front hairpiece: Before removing a lace-front hairpiece, dampen the lace with acetone or solvent in order to loosen it from the scalp (Figure 19). Do not pull or stretch the lace. To apply solvent, use a piece of cotton or a brush. After the

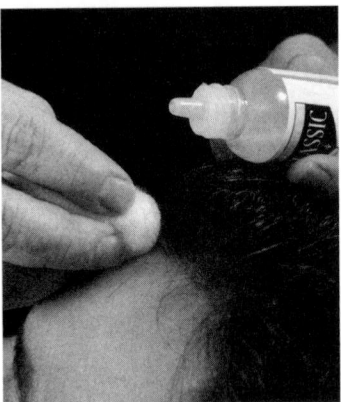

FIGURE 19 | Dampen lace with solvent to remove hairpiece.

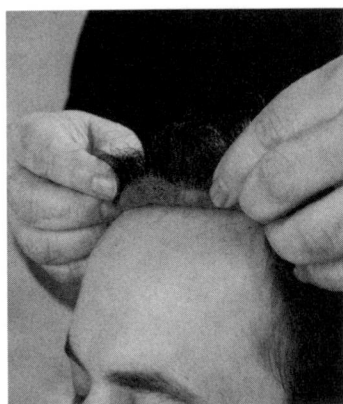

FIGURE 20 | Remove hairpiece gently.

lace becomes loosened, use the fingertips to remove the tape from the scalp (Figure 20). Do not pull off the hairpiece by tugging on the hair. Clean the reinforced areas with a small brush dipped in acetone or other solvent.

Partial Hairpieces

For a small degree of hair loss, a partial lace fill-in may be all that is required. Partial hairpieces can be made for the front or crown areas of the head. The measuring, application, and cutting techniques are the same as those used for full-hairpiece styles. Be sure that the area to be covered is shaved to facilitate better adherence of the spirit gum and hairpiece.

Facial Hairpieces

Facial hairpieces are attached with spirit gum. Mustaches, sideburns, and beards may all be attached in the same manner. Clean the facial area and apply spirit gum to the appropriate section. Wait until the gum is tacky, position the piece, and gently press down with a lint-free cloth. Trim the piece to the desired style.

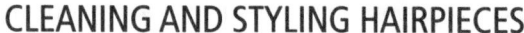 CLEANING AND STYLING HAIRPIECES

With the proper care, a well-constructed hairpiece will last for years. Manufacturers furnish instructions on the care of their hairpieces that both the barber and client should follow carefully. Clients should have at least two hairpieces to ensure that one will always be in good condition while the other one is being serviced and maintained.

▷ procedure no. 4

Cleaning Human Hair Hairpieces

Hairpieces must be kept clean just as natural hair must be kept clean. Cleaning should be performed carefully to help maintain the life of the hairpiece. Use the following guidelines and the manufacturer's recommendations to clean a hairpiece:

1. Remove all the old tape and clean any reinforced areas by dabbing them lightly with acetone or recommended solvent.

2. Put enough cleaner in a glass bowl so that the hairpiece can be submerged. Place the front of the hairpiece with the material side facing up into the solvent and allow to soak for three to five minutes. Swish the hairpiece back and forth (or dip it up and down) in the cleaner until all residue is removed from the hair and foundation.

3. With a small brush, gently tap the edge of the hairpiece until the adhesive has been removed. Do not rub or scrub.

4. If the solvent darkens, replace the cleaning agent until all residue is removed from the hair.

5   Place a towel on a flat surface and place the hairpiece with the material side facing upward on the towel.

6   Repeat the gum-removing procedure if any adhesive is left on the hairpiece.

7   If the adhesive forms a powder on the lace, place a little water on your fingertips and, in a sliding motion, allow the lace to absorb the water.

8   Gently press out the cleaner with the towel and allow to dry.

9   Fasten the dried hairpiece to the wig block with T-pins and comb out gently.

10 Set the piece in the desired style, cover with a hair net, and let it air-dry. Hairpieces may also be dried and styled with a blow-dryer while on the client's head. The scalp must be clean and dry and the hairpiece foundation thoroughly dried on a head mold before attaching it to the client's scalp. Moisten the hairpiece with a light water mist, being careful not to dampen the foundation. Style the hair as desired and cover with a styling hair net. Use the blow-dryer on a low, warm setting to dry the hair in place.

Cleaning Synthetic Hairpieces

Synthetic hairpieces should never be cleaned in solvent. Attach the hairpiece to a plastic foam head mold with T-pins. Then immerse it in lukewarm water with a mild shampoo. Do not use hot water, which would cause the hairpiece to shrink or become matted and tangled. Swish the hairpiece around in the shampoo solution. Rinse with clean, lukewarm water. Permit the hairpiece to dry naturally, pinned on the mold overnight; if time does not permit, place it under a dryer with cool air. Some hairpieces may be dry-cleaned, so always follow the manufacturer's instructions.

Basic Hairpiece Care

- Use the manufacturer's tape, antiseptic, cleaner, and softeners.

- When the hairpiece is not being worn, it should be placed on an appropriate block.

- Some hairpieces should be removed for showering and swimming.

- Clean the hairpiece after the first week of wear, and then every three to four weeks or as needed.

- Never fold the hairpiece.

- Always follow manufacturer's recommendations for removing the hairpiece.

- Apply light hair dressings and sprays sparingly and with even distribution.

- Set hairpieces with plain water.

Reconditioning Hairpieces

Reconditioning treatments should be given as often as necessary to prevent dryness or brittleness of the hair. Reconditioning treatments may also be used to liven up hairpieces that look dull and lifeless.

A small amount of reconditioner may be used, as directed by the manufacturer. If a slight color adjustment is necessary due to fading or yellowing, a suitable temporary color rinse is recommended. Select the rinse carefully so that the color matches that of the client's hair.

▷ procedure no. 5

Coloring Hairpieces

Permanent haircoloring products (aniline derivatives) can be used only on hairpieces made of 100 percent human hair. Use the following procedure and manufacturer's recommendations when coloring a hairpiece with permanent haircoloring products.

1. The hairpiece is first cleaned with a dry-cleaning solvent.

2. Cover the head form block with plastic material to prevent staining from the coloring product.

3. Secure the hairpiece firmly with T-pins or straight pins in the front, back, and sides.

4. Perform a strand test on a small section of hair to determine the color desired. If using a tint with peroxide, apply it on a dry hair strand.

5. Mix the haircoloring of desired shade.

6. Apply with a haircoloring brush.

7. Comb the color product through lightly, being careful not to saturate the foundation.

8. Test every five minutes until the desired shade is obtained.

9. After processing, rinse thoroughly with warm water. Shampoo and condition according to manufacturer's directions.

10. Comb and set into the desired style.

▷ procedure no. 6

Permanent Waving Hairpieces

Permanent waving a hairpiece requires time, creativity, and careful attention to detail. The objective is to create a natural look, so the hairpiece should be custom wrapped according to the contours of the head and the flow of the hair sewn into the hairpiece.

The rod placement does not rest on the scalp of the hairpiece as it would in a perm procedure on natural hair. Instead, the rods are floated to eliminate weight and rod marks on the base. Floating is accomplished by using T-pins to support the rod above the base of the hairpiece. The pins are inserted at both ends of the rod and are held in place by the rubber band of the perm rod. When the hairpiece has been rodded and secured with the T-pins, the procedure for completing the perming process is as follows:

1   Select a mild permanent wave solution appropriate for bleached or damaged hair types. Hold the wig block upside down and rotate while applying the solution. Allow the excess solution to drip into the sink before setting the block back on the stand.

2   Take a test curl every minute until processing is complete.

3   Rinse the hairpiece for 10 to 15 minutes. The hairpiece will be air neutralized and does not require the application of a neutralizing solution.

4   Thoroughly blot each rod with paper towels to absorb as much water as possible.

5   Remove the T-pins and hang the block upside down. Leave the rods in the hairpiece and cover with a plastic cap for 24 hours.

6   On day two, remove the cap and allow the piece to dry for another day. Remove the rods only when the hair is completely dry.

General Recommendations and Reminders

▫ Comb hairpieces carefully to avoid matting, loss of hair, or damage.

◘ Use a wide-tooth comb to avoid weakening or damaging the foundation.

◘ Never rub or wring cleaning fluids from the hairpiece. Let it dry naturally.

◘ Be careful not to cut too much hair when cutting, tapering, and blending a hairpiece.

◘ Take accurate measurements to assure a comfortable and secure fit.

◘ Recondition hairpieces as often as necessary to prevent dryness, brittleness, or dullness of the hair.

◘ If required by the manufacturer, dry-clean hairpieces before styling.

◘ Brush and comb hairpieces with a downward movement.

◘ To avoid damage to the foundation, never lighten or cold-wave a hairpiece.

◘ If coloring is necessary, it must be done with care.

■ TECH TERM

A cold wave is an alkaline permanent wave solution that does not require heat to process.

Full Wigs

Although most men might not choose to wear a full wig, many women enjoy the coverage, convenience, and instant style changes they can achieve with wigs. Ready-to-wear wigs are usually made of modacrylic fibers such as Kanekalon, Dynel, and venicelon.

Construction and Fit

Full, ready-made wigs are constructed on a stretch cap made of lightweight elastic. The wig has permanent elastic bands at the sides designed to hold it in place. It should fit comfortably, but tightly enough to maintain its position without slipping, shifting, or lifting. Wigs come in a wide variety of colors and in many different styles.

▷ procedure no. 7

Cleaning Wigs

Cleaning ready-made wigs is a fairly quick and easy process. Use the guidelines provided and the manufacturer's cleaning instructions to clean ready-made wigs.

1. Brush the wig thoroughly to remove all surface dirt and residue.

2. Mix a solution of warm water and mild shampoo in a bowl.

3. Dip the entire wig into the solution; swish it around in the solution.

4. Rinse the wig in clean, cold water.

5. Blot it dry with a towel.

6. Turn the wig inside out and dry it with a towel.

7. Pin the wig to a head mold or wig block of the correct size.

8. Carefully brush the hair into place.

9. Permit the wig to dry naturally, pinned to the form.

10. If necessary, use cool air to dry it quickly.

11. When dry, brush it into the proper style.

Selling Nonsurgical Hair Replacements

In order to sell men's hairpiece replacements, it is important to know why men buy them. In the first part of this section, the results of a study concerning the perceptions of bald and balding men were discussed. When a man expresses an interest in wearing a nonsurgical hair replacement to his barber, he won't appreciate a hard-sell approach. His interest has already been made evident and he is simply looking for guidance and purchasing information at this stage. It is the barber's responsibility to educate the client about the possibilities and options available to him.

Just as a hard-sell approach should be avoided, the barber should never promise what cannot be delivered nor raise the client's expectations to an unreasonable level. For example, it is not professionally ethical to convince an elderly man that he can recapture the appearance of his 40s with a nonsurgical hair replacement. It simply cannot be done. The color of the nonsurgical hair replacement is also an important consideration. Dark, opaque colors are not recommended for any age group, especially older persons. It is better to recommend a salt-and-pepper blend or medium-brown shade. The more natural looking the color, the less obvious the hairpiece will appear.

Marketing Techniques

- *Hairpiece display:* One or two correctly styled hairpieces displayed in the shop will alert clients to the fact that nonsurgical hair replacement services are performed there. Make certain that the sample is clean and nicely styled. It should be large enough to cover the average balding area of a man, as most clients will be men with an average amount of hair loss, and many may want to try it on.

  NOTE: *Be sure to sanitize the hairpiece after each client.*

- *Referrals and word-of-mouth:* These two methods may be a slower approach, and are not to be relied on exclusively for new business, but they are still very effective forms of advertising. Personal referrals are the best evidence of pleased and satisfied clients.

- *Window displays:* Window displays can add to increased hairpiece sales. Before-and-after illustrations in the shop window let the walk-by and drive-by traffic know that nonsurgical hair replacements can be obtained through the barbershop. It can also offer encouragement to those clients whom you feel cannot be approached directly with the idea of wearing a hairpiece. As they become more comfortable with the idea of a hairpiece, or see other men in the shop receiving nonsurgical hair replacement services, they may feel more inclined to explore their own options.

◻ *Personal approach:* The personal approach may certainly be used to suggest a hairpiece to a client; however, it must be a tactful approach. Wait for an opening during the consultation or haircut service when the client brings up his hair loss condition in the conversation and offer him the opportunity to try on a hairpiece. A quick demonstration may convince him of his improved appearance and lead to a sale.

◻ *Print ads:* Print ads include all printed advertising, from coupons to billboards. It is important to advertise nonsurgical hair replacement services because not all barbershops pursue this market. In many areas an extra line in the telephone book that mentions nonsurgical hair replacements will pay for itself. Your phone book also may contain a special listing for hair goods. This is another good classification in the phone directory to place an advertisement.

In some communities, newspaper advertising is inexpensive and profitable. If a model is used, be sure to secure a model release for any photos that might be used in the ads. Even if the model is your best friend, do not assume that a release is unnecessary.

◻ *Personal experience:* If you wear a hairpiece yourself, you can develop an excellent promotional approach. Often, nothing is more convincing than your own before-and-after demonstration. The fact that you wear a hairpiece with assurance and complete ease can make a very strong impression on prospective hairpiece clients.

ALTERNATIVE HAIR RESTORATION TECHNIQUES

In addition to nonsurgical hair replacements, three other approaches to hair restoration are available for men. The first are *medicinal drugs* known as minoxidil and finasteride, which are known by different brand names depending on the manufacturer. The second is *surgery,* which includes procedures such as hair transplantation, scalp reduction, and flap surgery. A third option is the *hair weave.*

Hair Restoration Medicinal Drugs

A 2 percent solution of minoxidil applied twice daily has been shown to be moderately effective for about 50 percent of the men using it. Clinical studies conducted by Pharmacia and Up-john (the maker, recently acquired by Pfizer, of the Rogaine brand minoxidil) revealed that 26 percent of the men reported average to dense hair growth and 33 percent reported minimal hair growth after four months of treatment with Rogaine. Minoxidil is available for both men and women and in two different strengths: 2 percent regular and 5 percent extra-strength formula.

Surgical Hair Restoration

The three types of surgical hair restoration available are hair transplants, scalp reduction, and flap surgery.

- *Hair transplantation* is strictly a medical procedure that should be performed only by licensed medical

i **FYI**

Finasteride is an oral prescription medication for men only that provides them with an additional hair restoration option. Although it is considered more effective and convenient than minoxidil, its possible side effects include weight gain and loss of sexual function.

professionals. The process consists of removing hair from normal areas of the scalp, such as the back and sides, and transplanting it into the bald areas under a local anesthetic. Small sections of hair from single strands to larger plugs of 7 to 10 hairs are surgically removed, including the hair follicle, papilla, and hair bulb, and reset in the bald area. With today's technological advances in hair restoration, micrographs have replaced the larger "plug" sections of the past few decades. The transplanted hair usually grows normally in its new environment while the area from which the hair was removed heals and shrinks in size to a very tiny scar.

- The surgeon must select the hair to be transplanted with care, taking into consideration color, texture, and type. Placement of the hair in the direction of natural growth to permit proper care and complimentary styling is also an important factor. Transplanted hair can last a lifetime if the service is performed properly. If the doctor is skilled and the individual cares for the hair as directed, hair transplants can be very successful as a method of permanently eliminating baldness.

- *Scalp reduction* is a process by which the bald area is removed from the scalp and surrounding scalp areas with hair growth are pulled together to fill in the spot.

- *Flap surgery,* like scalp reduction surgery, removes the bald scalp area. A flap of hair-bearing skin is then attached to what was the bald area.

Hair Weaves

The use of hair weaves, a form of nonsurgical hair replacement, has been practiced in barbershops for many years. Though numerous claims of new techniques and exclusive methods in hair weaving exist, the usual procedure consists of sewing or weaving a foundation onto the remaining hair at the scalp, and then weaving wefts of human hair to the foundation.

Because the foundation is attached to the remaining hair on the head, the foundation tends to move out from the scalp as the natural hair grows. Continual adjustments are required to maintain the desired appearance. The foundation must be tightened and brought close to the scalp every four to eight weeks depending on the rate of natural hair growth. The hair must be shampooed carefully in sections to avoid pulling and causing damage to the foundation or pain to the client. And, as with natural hair, it should receive periodic conditioning treatments to add luster and avoid dryness and damage.

THE NEXT STEP

As we have seen, many hair restoration options are available today. These options offer your clients the opportunity to improve their personal appearance and boost their self-confidence. However, hair restoration isn't the only way to improve one's appearance. A subtle or dramatic hair color change can also do the trick. In the next section, you will learn the basics of providing hair coloring and lightening services to your clients in a safe and professional manner.

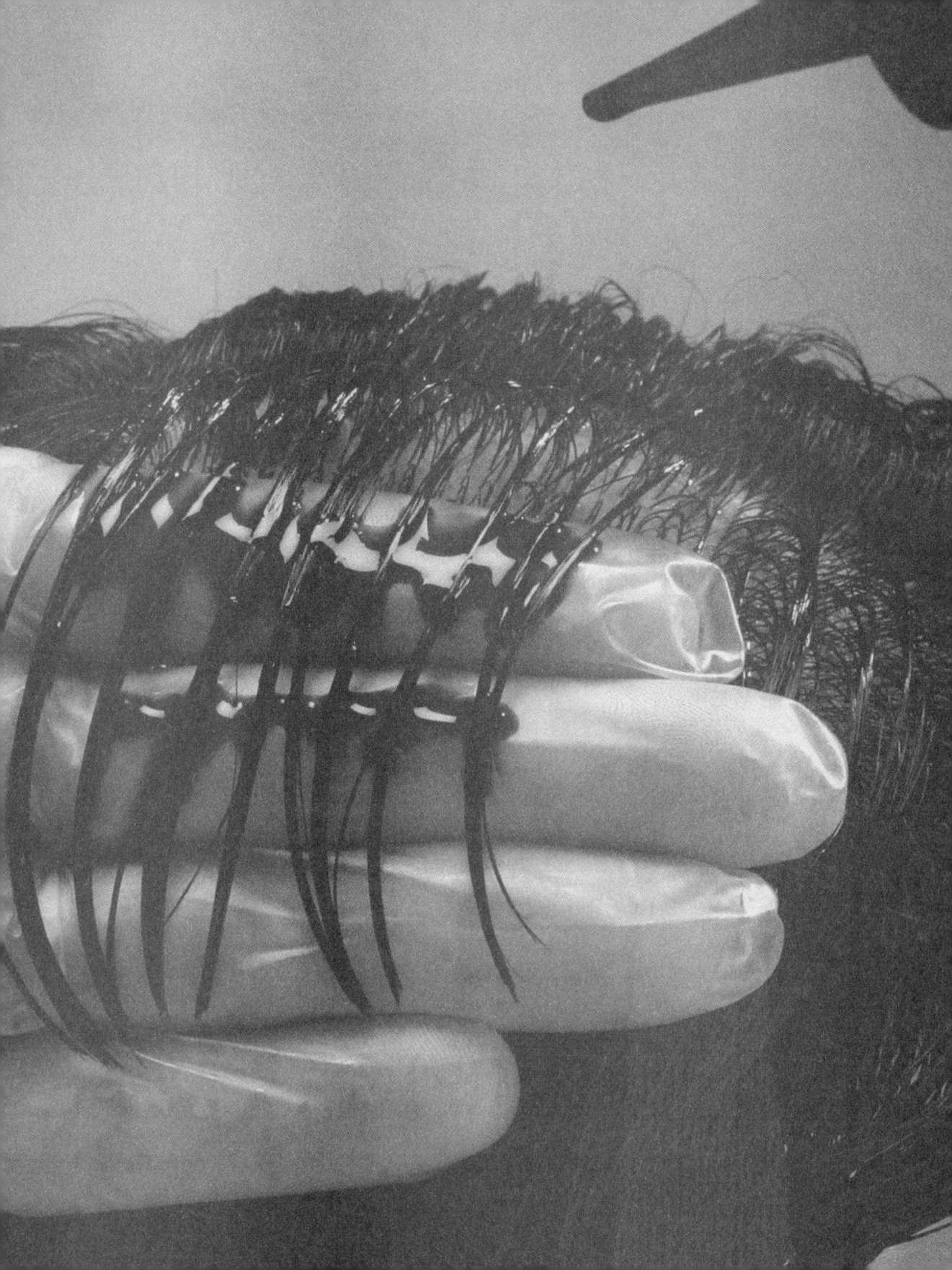

HAIRCOLORING AND LIGHTENING

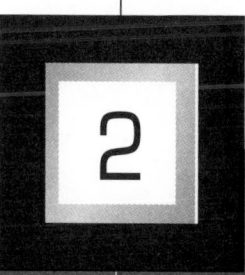

2

Men and women have altered their hair color for thousands of years. Early cultures considered colors to be symbols of power and mysticism. This belief led to body painting and haircoloring agents derived from vegetable and mineral dyes, as evidenced by chemicals and tools found in Egyptian tombs.

In the 1880s, American men had their beards and mustaches dyed in barbershops with coloring products that left the hair with strange iridescent tones or purple hues. These early formulations were made of silver nitrate, gold chloride and/or gum, and distilled water. Since the first synthetic dyes were developed in 1883, color technology and haircoloring processes have steadily improved in performance and safety.

Haircoloring is the science and art of changing the color of the hair. *Hair lightening* is the partial or total removal of natural pigment or artificial color from the hair. Haircoloring and lightening services offer the skillful barber yet another opportunity for building a loyal and lucrative clientele base.

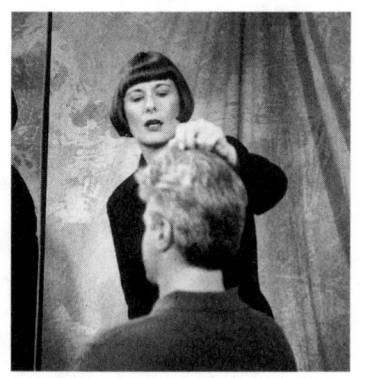

FIGURE 21 | Many clients choose to cover or blend gray hair.

Many shop clients will express an interest in haircolor at some point or another. Clients who enjoy fashion changes, are prematurely gray, or wish to maintain a youthful appearance represent typical haircoloring service clients (Figure 21). Others may wish to change the natural color of their hair to a more attractive shade or to create decorative effects, such as highlighting or streaking.

Barbers who want to provide successful haircoloring and lightening services to their clients need to understand hair structure, the laws of color, and the processes associated with color and lightening products. A skilled haircolorist is proficient in adding artificial pigment to natural, previously colored, or prelightened hair and understands the process of diffusing natural pigment through lightening agents.

CHARACTERISTICS AND STRUCTURE OF HAIR

The client's hair structure will affect the quality and ultimate success of the haircolor service. The strength of the cuticle and the amount of elasticity and natural pigment in the cortex are important considerations in determining haircoloring options and product selection. Other hair structure factors relevant to a haircoloring or lightening service include texture, density, porosity, and natural color.

- *Texture:* The diameter of the individual hair strand determines whether the hair texture is classified as fine, medium, or coarse. Melanin is distributed differently within the different textures. Melanin granules in fine hair are grouped tightly, so the hair takes color faster and may appear darker. Medium-textured hair has an average response time to haircolor products, and coarse hair may take longer to process (Figure 22).

- *Density:* To assure proper coverage, the density of the hair should be taken into account when applying haircolor or lighteners.

- *Porosity:* The porosity level of the hair influences its ability to absorb liquids. Porous hair accepts haircolor products faster and permits a darker saturation than less porous hair. Hair with a low porosity level has a tight cuticle that makes it resistant to moisture and chemical penetration, with the result that it can require a longer processing time. In hair that has an average porosity level, the cuticle is slightly raised and the hair tends to process in an average amount of time. High porosity is indicated by a lifted cuticle. Such hair may take color quickly but it may also fade

■ TECH TERM

The *cortex* is the middle layer of the hair shaft.

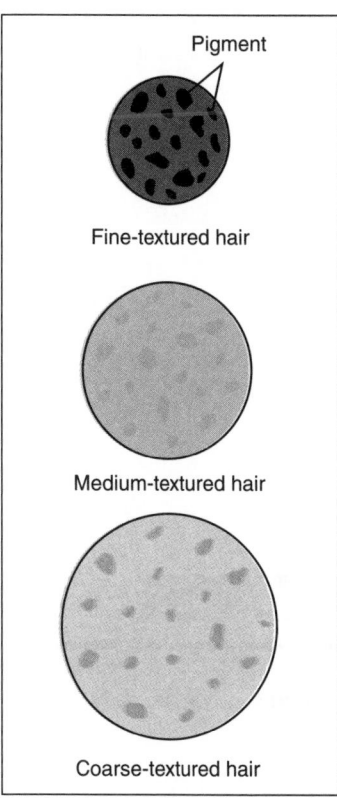

FIGURE 22 | Melanin distribution according to hair texture.

■ TECH TERM

Melanin is the coloring matter or pigment of the skin and hair.

sooner than other porosity levels, due to an inability to hold the color for the normal amount of time.

☐ *Natural color:* Natural hair color ranges from black to dark brown to red, and from dark blond to lightest blond. Eumelanin gives black and brown color to hair and pheomelanin is the melanin found in yellowish-blond, ginger, and red tones. The three factors that determine all natural colors, from jet black to light blond, are the thickness of the hair, the total number and size of pigment granules, and the ratio of eumelanin to pheomelanin. White hair is actually the color of keratin without the influence of melanin and therefore does not contain either type.

☐ *Contributing pigment* is the pigment that lies under the natural hair color. The foundation of haircoloring is based on modifying this pigment with haircoloring products to create new pigments or colors.

Gray hair is normally associated with aging, although heredity is also a contributing factor. In most cases, the loss of pigment increases as a person ages, resulting in a range of gray tones from blended to solid. The amount of gray in an individual's hair is measured in percentages, as presented in Table 1, and

Table 1	DETERMINING THE PERCENTAGE OF GRAY HAIR

PERCENTAGE OF GRAY HAIR	CHARACTERISTICS
30%	More pigmented than gray hair
50%	Even mixture of gray and pigmented hair
70 to 90%	More gray than pigmented; most of remaining pigment is located at the back of the head
100%	Virtually no pigmented hair; tends to look white

requires special care when formulating haircolor applications. (The challenges and solutions associated with coloring gray hair are discussed later in this section.)

■ | COLOR THEORY

Color is a form of visible light energy. Although the human eye sees only six basic colors, the brain is capable of visualizing the combinations of different wavelengths relevant to the three primary and three secondary colors. The movement of light rays that are absorbed or reflected by natural hair pigment or artificial pigment added to the hair creates the colors we see.

The Laws of Color

The laws of color regulate the mixing of dyes and pigment to make other colors. They are based in science and adapted to art. The laws of color serve as guidelines for harmonious color mixing. For example, equal parts of red and blue mixed together always make violet.

Primary Colors

Primary colors are basic or true colors that cannot be created by combining other colors. The three primary colors are yellow, red, and blue (Figure 23). All other colors are created by some combination of red, yellow, or blue. Colors with a predominance of blue are cool-toned colors and colors that are predominantly red are warm-toned colors.

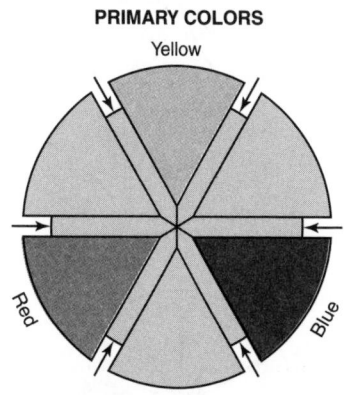

PRIMARY COLORS

FIGURE 23 | Primary colors.

- ■ Blue is the darkest and only cool primary color. Blue creates depth or darkness in any color to which it is added.

- ■ Red is the medium primary color. When added to blue-based colors, red makes them appear lighter.

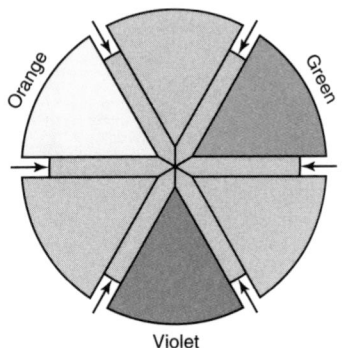

FIGURE 24 | Secondary colors.

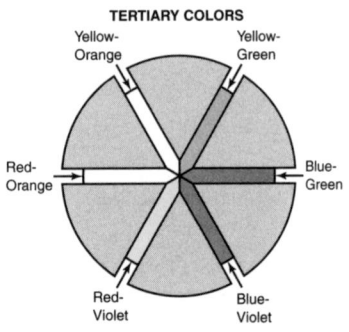

FIGURE 25 | Tertiary colors.

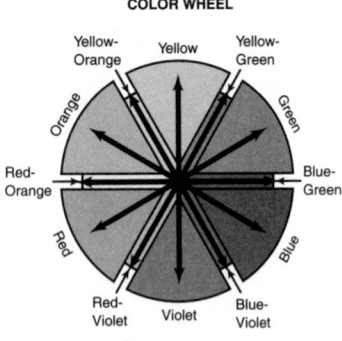

FIGURE 26 | Complementary colors.

Conversely, red added to a yellow color will cause it to become darker.

☐ Yellow is the lightest of the primary colors and will lighten and brighten other colors.

Secondary Colors

Secondary colors are created by mixing equal amounts of two primary colors. Mixed in equal parts, yellow and blue create green, blue and red create violet, and red and yellow create orange (Figure 24). Natural hair color is made up of a combination of primary and secondary colors.

Tertiary Colors

Tertiary colors are created by mixing equal amounts of one primary color with one of its adjacent secondary colors. Presented in their order on the color wheel, tertiary colors are yellow-green, blue-green, blue-violet, red-violet, red-orange, and yellow-orange (Figure 25).

Note: Quaternary colors are all other combinations of all three primary colors.

Complementary Colors

Complementary colors are any two colors situated directly across from each other on the color wheel (Figure 26). When mixed together their action is to neutralize each other. For example, when mixed in equal amounts, red and green neutralize each other, creating brown. Orange and blue neutralize each other, and yellow and violet neutralize each other.

Complementary colors are always composed of a primary and a secondary color, and complementary pairs always consist of all three primary colors. For example, the color wheel shows that the complement of red (a primary color) is green (a secondary color). Green is made up of blue and yellow (both primary colors). So, all three primary colors are represented to varying degrees in the complementary pair of red and green.

Tone or Hue of Color

The tone or hue is the basic name of a color, such as red, yellow, blue-green, and so on. Tone is also used to describe the warmth or coolness of a color. The warm colors, also known as high-lighting colors, are red, orange, and yellow. The cool colors, also known as ash or drab, are blue, green, and violet.

Level

The level of color is the density of a color and indicates the degree of lightness or darkness of a color. Colors lighten when mixed with white and darken when mixed with black. In hair-coloring, the Level System is used to analyze the lightness or darkness of a hair color. Hair colors, both natural and color-treated, are arranged on a scale of 1 to 10, with 1 being black and 10 indicating lightest blond (Figure 27). The Level System is crucial to formulating, matching, and correcting colors.

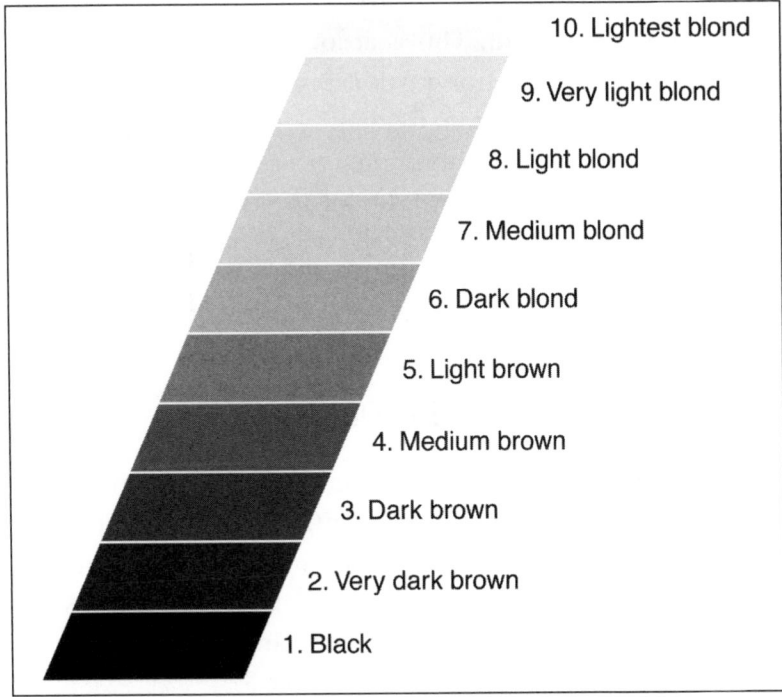

10. Lightest blond

9. Very light blond

8. Light blond

7. Medium blond

6. Dark blond

5. Light brown

4. Medium brown

3. Dark brown

2. Very dark brown

1. Black

FIGURE 27 │ The Level System.

Saturation

Saturation, or intensity, refers to the degree of concentration or amount of pigment in the color. It is the strength of a color. For example, a saturated red is very vivid. Any color can be more or less saturated. The more saturated the product, the more dramatic the change in hair color.

Base Color

Artificial haircolors are developed from primary and secondary colors to form base colors. A base color is the predominant tone of a color, which greatly influences the final color result. For example, a violet base color will produce cool results and help to minimize yellow tones. Blue base colors minimize orange tones, and a red-orange base creates warm, bright tones in the hair.

Identifying Natural Level and Tone

The first step in performing a haircolor service is to identify the natural level of the hair. This is accomplished by holding the manufacturer's swatches or a color ring up to the client's hair for matching. It is important to identify the natural level of the hair so that an accurate determination can be made as to what the final hair color results will look like. These results will be based on the combination of the natural hair color and the artificial color that is added to it.

 ## HAIRCOLORING PRODUCTS

Haircoloring products generally fall into four classifications: temporary, semipermanent, demipermanent, and permanent (Table 2). These classifications indicate color fastness, or its ability to remain on the hair, and are determined by the chemical composition and molecular weight of the pigments and dyes within the products (Table 3).

Table 2	REVIEW OF HAIRCOLOR CATEGORIES AND THEIR USES

CATEGORY	USES
Temporary color	Creates subtle color change Shampoos from the hair Neutralizes yellow hair
Semipermanent color	Introduces a client to haircolor services Adds subtle color results Tones prelightened hair
Demipermanent color	Blends gray hair Enhances natural color Tones prelightened hair Refreshes faded color Filler in color correction
Permanent haircolor	Changes existing haircolor Covers gray Creates bright or natural-looking haircolor changes

Temporary Haircolor (Nonoxidation Color)

Temporary colors utilize pigment and dye molecules of the greatest molecular weight, making these molecules the largest in the four classifications of hair color. The large size of the color molecule prevents penetration into the cuticle layer, producing only a coating action on the outside of the strand. This coating action usually results in very subtle color changes, lasting only until the next shampoo (Figure 28).

The chemical composition of a temporary color is acidic in reaction, creating a physical change rather than a chemical change in the hair shaft. As a result, patch tests are not required when applying temporary color. Temporary rinses have a pH range of 2.0 to 4.5.

■ TECH TERM

A *nonoxidation color* promotes a temporary or semipermanent change in haircolor through either a coating action or self-penetrating action without the use of an oxidizer, such as hydrogen peroxide.

Table 3	**FOUR CLASSIFICATIONS OF COLOR**			

CHARACTERISTIC	TEMPORARY	SEMIPERMANENT	DEMIPERMANENT	PERMANENT
Molecular weight of dye molecule	Large	Medium	Medium-small	Small
pH	Acid	Slightly alkaline	Moderately alkaline	Alkaline
Reaction or change	Physical	Chemical & physical	Chemical & physical	Chemical & physical
Color fastness	Removed with shampooing	Fades gradually	Fades slower than semipermanent color	Permanent
Color changes	Deposits	Deposits	No-lift, Deposit only	Lifts and deposits

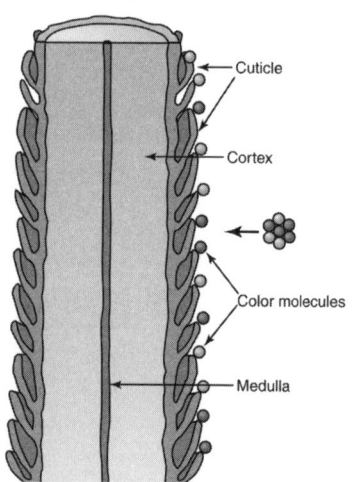

FIGURE 28 | Action of temporary haircolor.

Cuticle
Cortex
Color molecules
Medulla

TECH TERM

A *certified color* is a commercial coloring product permitted in foods, drugs, and cosmetics by the FDA.

Types of Temporary Haircolor

- *Color rinses* are used to highlight the color or add color to the hair. These rinses contain certified colors and remain on the hair until the next shampoo. Two types of color rinses are available: instant and concentrated. Instant rinses are applied straight from the bottle and remain in the hair. Concentrated rinses are mixed with hot water before application, processed for 5 to 10 minutes, and then rinsed. Both types of rinses may leave traces of the darker shades on combs, brushes, and clothing.

- *Color-enhancing shampoos* combine the action of a color rinse with that of a shampoo. These shampoos generally contain certified colors, produce highlights, and impart slight color tones to the hair.

- *Crayons* are sticks of coloring compounded with soaps or synthetic waxes. They are sometimes used to color gray or white hair between hair tint retouches.

Crayons are often used by men as a temporary coloring for mustaches. They are available in several standard colors: blond; light, medium, and dark brown; black; and auburn.

◻ *Haircolor sprays* are applied to dry hair from aerosol containers. Color sprays are usually available in vibrant colors and are generally used for special or party effects.

◻ *Haircolor mousses and gels* combine slight color and styling effects in one product.

Semipermanent Haircolor (Nonoxidation Color)

Traditional semipermanent haircolor products are also known as *direct dyes* because they do not develop color. Semipermanent pigment molecules are of a lesser molecular weight than those of temporary colors. This facilitates the physical capability to partially penetrate into the cortex. Although some color does enter the cortex, most of the pigment molecules stain the cuticle layer through absorption. These molecules are also small enough to diffuse out of the hair during shampooing and tend to fade with each shampoo. Most semipermanent colors will last from six to eight shampoos (Figure 29).

The chemical composition of semipermanent color is mildly alkaline in reaction, causes the cortex to swell, and raises the cuticle to allow some penetration. This chemical composition combines small color molecules, solvents, alkaline swelling agents, and surfactants to create a type of color that is known as self-penetrating. Self-penetrating colors tend to make a mild chemical change as well as a physical change.

Most semipermanent colors do not contain ammonia and may be used right out of the bottle. Although normally gentle on the hair, semipermanent colors require a patch test prior to application to prevent the occurrence of product sensitivity or allergic reaction.

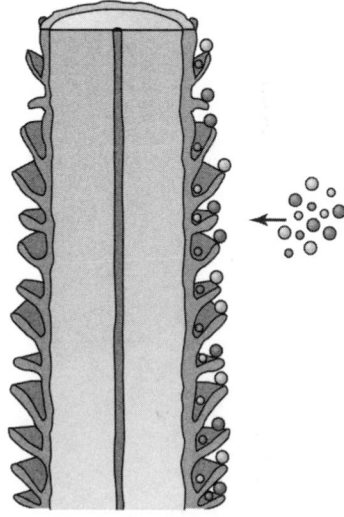

FIGURE 29 │ Action of semipermanent haircolor.

■ TECH TERM

A *surfactant* is a base detergent.

Semipermanent haircolors typically fall within the 7.0 to 9.0 pH range; however, some formulations use salt bonds to improve colorfastness and may range between 7.0 and 8.0 on the pH scale. Due to the slight alkalinity of semipermanent color, these haircolor services should be followed with a mild, acid-balanced shampoo and conditioning. This will neutralize any residual alkalinity and help to restore the hair to normal pH levels.

Semipermanent haircolor may be used to:

- cover or blend partially gray hair without affecting its natural color (most semipermanent colors are designed to cover hair that is no more than 25 percent gray)

- highlight, enhance, or deepen color tones in the hair

- serve as a nonperoxide toner for prelighted hair

Demipermanent Haircolor (Oxidation Color)

■ TECH TERM

Oxidation color color developed from a chemical reaction that combines an element or compound with oxygen to produce an oxide.

■ TECH TERM

A *developer* is an oxidizing agent, usually hydrogen peroxide, used to develop color. An *activator* is an additive used to quicken the action or progress of hydrogen peroxide.

Demipermanent haircolor, also known as *no-lift, deposit-only haircolor* (referred to as semipermanent by some manufacturers), is longer lasting than traditional semipermanent color. These products are designed to deposit color without lifting (lightening) natural or artificial color in the hair and are considered a type of oxidation color. As such, they are not used directly out of the bottle but must be mixed with a low-volume developer or activator immediately before use. The oxidizing agent in the developer causes an oxidation reaction, which develops the color (Figure 30).

Demipermanent and other deposit-only colors darken the natural color of hair when applied. They are available in gel, cream, or liquid forms and require a patch test before application.

Demipermanent haircolor may be used to:

- impart vivid color results.

- cover nonpigmented hair.

- refresh faded permanent color.

- deposit tonal changes without lift.
- reverse highlight.
- perform corrective coloring.

Permanent Haircolor (Oxidation Color)

Permanent haircolor is mixed with a developer (hydrogen peroxide) and remains in the hair shaft. When the hair grows, a touch-up or retouch application is required to blend the color of the previously colored hair with the new hair growth. Permanent haircolor products usually contain ammonia, oxidative tints, and peroxide and require a patch test.

Permanent haircolor products can lighten and deposit color in one process. They can lighten natural hair color because they are more alkaline than demipermanent oxidation colors and are usually mixed with a higher-volume developer. The amount of lift is controlled by the pH of the color and the concentration of peroxide in the developer. As the pH of the color and concentration increase, the amount of lift increases as well. Permanent haircolor products are usually mixed with an equal amount of 20-volume peroxide and are capable of lifting one or two levels. When mixed with higher volumes of peroxide, permanent colors can lift up to four levels. Because some manufacturers recommend a 2:1 ratio of developer to haircolor, always read the manufacturer's directions. Permanent hair color should not be applied immediately following a permanent wave process.

Permanent haircolor is considered a penetrating tint because after the tint is mixed with an oxidizer it has the ability to penetrate through the cuticle into the cortex of the hair shaft. This action is facilitated by aniline derivatives that diffuse into the cortex and then form larger permanent tint molecules that become trapped within the cortex. In this way, the cortex undergoes permanent chemical and structural changes (Figure 31).

Permanent tints are alkaline in reaction and generally range between 9.0 and 10.5 on the pH scale. After processing,

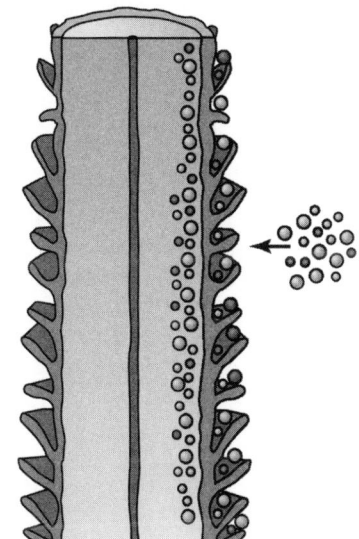

FIGURE 30 | Action of demipermanent haircolor.

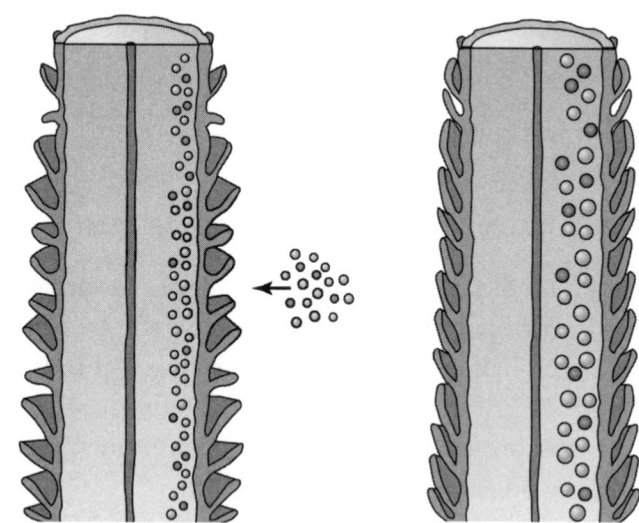

FIGURE 31 | Action of permanent haircolor.

the hair is shampooed and as it dries it begins to return to its normal pH. This causes the cortex to shrink and the cuticle to close. Both actions tend to further trap the color molecules. Except for residual color product following the haircolor application, permanent haircolor does not wash out during the shampoo process. Eventually the color will fade and may require refreshing. When new growth occurs, a line of demarcation will develop between the old and new growth and will require a retouch.

Permanent haircoloring products are generally regarded as the best products for covering gray hair. This is because they simultaneously remove natural pigment through the action of lifting while adding artificial color to both the gray and pigmented hair.

Types of Permanent Haircolor

Permanent haircolors fall into four classifications: oxidation tints, vegetable tints, metallic or mineral dyes, and compound dyes.

OXIDATION TINTS Oxidation tints are also known as aniline derivative tints, penetrating tints, synthetic-organic tints, and amino tints. Oxidation tints can lighten and deposit color in a single process and are available in a wide variety of colors. *Toners* also fall into the category of permanent color. Toners are aniline derivative products of pale, delicate shades designed for use on prelightened hair.

Most oxidation tints contain aniline derivatives and require a predisposition (patch) test before the service is performed. As long as the hair is of normal strength and kept in good condition, oxidation tints are compatible with other professional chemical services.

Oxidation tints are sold in bottles, canisters, and tubes, in either a semiliquid or cream form. These products must be mixed with hydrogen peroxide, which activates the chemical reaction known as oxidation. This reaction begins as soon as the two compounds are combined, so the mixed tint must be used immediately. Any leftover tint must be discarded because it deteriorates quickly.

Timing the application of the tint depends upon the product and the volume of peroxide selected. Consult the manufacturer's directions for assistance. A strand test should always be performed to ensure satisfactory results.

VEGETABLE TINTS Vegetable tints are haircoloring products made from various plants, such as herbs and flowers. In the past, indigo, chamomile, sage, Egyptian henna, and other plants were used to color the hair. Henna is still used as a professional haircoloring product, but should be used with some caution. Henna has a coating action that can build up with overuse and prevent the penetration of other chemicals. Henna also penetrates the cortex and attaches to the salt bonds. Both of these actions may leave the hair unfit for other professional treatments. Even though vegetable tints are considered permanent, they are nonoxidation color products.

METALLIC OR MINERAL DYES Metallic dyes are advertised as color restorers or progressive colors. The metallic ingredients, such as lead acetate or silver nitrate, react with the keratin in the hair, turning it brown. This reaction creates a colored film coating that produces a dull metallic appearance. Repeated treatments damage the hair and can react adversely with many professional chemical services. Metallic dyes are not professional coloring products.

COMPOUND DYES Compound dyes are metallic or mineral dyes combined with a vegetable tint. The metallic salts are added to give the product more staying power and to create different colors. Like metallic dyes, compound dyes are not used professionally.

Hydrogen Peroxide Developers

A developer is an oxidizing agent that supplies oxygen gas for the development of color molecules when mixed with an oxidative haircolor product. This action creates a color change in the hair when the oxidizer combines with the melanin in the hair. Most developers range between 2.5 and 4.5 on the pH scale.

Hydrogen peroxide (H_2O_2) serves as the primary oxidizing agent used in haircoloring. As the oxygen and melanin combine, the peroxide solution begins to diffuse and lighten the melanin within the cortex. The smaller structure and spread-out distribution of the diffused melanin gives the hair a lighter appearance. This diffused melanin is called oxymelanin.

In its purest form, hydrogen peroxide has a pH level of about 7.0. When diluted with water and other substances for use in haircoloring, hydrogen peroxide has a mild acidic pH of 3.5 to 4.0.

Strengths of Hydrogen Peroxide

Hydrogen peroxide alone produces a relatively mild lightening of the hair color and causes little damage to the hair shaft. When very pale shades are desired, however, further lightening must occur and a longer processing time or the mixture of a stronger formula is required.

In the scientific world, different strengths of hydrogen peroxide are identified as percentages. In haircoloring, the term *volume* is used to denote the different strengths of hydrogen peroxide (Table 4).

Volume is the measure of the potential oxidation of varying strengths of hydrogen peroxide. The lower the volume, the less lift is achieved; the higher the volume, the greater the lifting action.

Permanent haircolor products use 10-, 20-, 30-, or 40-volume hydrogen peroxide for proper color development. A 10-volume solution is recommended when less lightening is desired for color enhancement. The majority of permanent coloring products use 20-volume hydrogen peroxide for proper color development and to cover gray. A 30-volume developer is used to achieve additional lift and 40-volume is used with most high-lift colors to provide maximum lift in one step.

Hydrogen peroxide is distributed for use under a variety of names, such as *developer, oxidizer, generator,* and *catalyst.* Regardless of the name used, hydrogen peroxide is available in three forms: dry, cream, and liquid.

- ◻ *Dry peroxide,* in either tablet or powder form, is dissolved in liquid hydrogen peroxide to boost the

| Table 4 | PERCENTAGES AND VOLUMES OF HYDROGEN PEROXIDE |

PERCENTAGE OF H_2O_2 IN WATER	VOLUME OF OXYGEN SET FREE
1.5%	5
3%	10
6%	20
9%	30
12%	40

volume. The availability of liquid peroxide in a variety of volumes has made this product somewhat obsolete.

☐ *Cream peroxides* contain additives such as thickeners, drabbers, conditioners, and acids for stabilization. The thickeners help to create a product that tends to stay moist on the hair longer than liquid peroxide, is easy to control, and prevents dripping during the brush-and-bowl method of application.

NOTE: Additives may dilute the strength of the formula and make it undesirable when full strength is needed.

☐ *Liquid hydrogen peroxide* contains a stabilizing acid that brings the pH to 3.5–4.0. This form of peroxide is convenient because it can be used with most of today's bleach and tint formulas.

Hydrogen Peroxide Safety Precautions

☐ Use clean implements when measuring, using, and storing hydrogen peroxide. Even a small amount of dirt or impurities can cause hydrogen peroxide to deteriorate.

☐ Never measure the needed amount of hydrogen peroxide by pouring it into the lid of another product. The residue will cause the product in the container to oxidize as it sits on the shelf and render it unusable.

☐ Do not allow hydrogen peroxide formulations to come in contact with metal. Metal causes the oxidation process to occur too quickly to allow proper color development.

☐ Avoid breathing in vapors caused by mixing hydrogen peroxide and haircolor products.

☐ A hydrogen peroxide volume of 20 or more can cause skin irritations, chemical burns, and hair damage.

Activators

An activator is an oxidizer that is added to hydrogen peroxide for the purpose of increasing its chemical action. This results in an increased lifting power, which is controlled by the number of activators that are added to the peroxide. Up to three activators can be used for on-the-scalp applications, and up to four for off-the-scalp processes.

Lighteners

Lighteners are chemical compounds that lighten hair by dispersing, dissolving, and decolorizing the natural or artificial hair pigment (Figure 32). This is accomplished through the use of a bleach formula, hydrogen peroxide, and the chemical heat produced by the combination of these ingredients. When mixed for use, the pH of lighteners is around 10.0 on the pH scale.

The hair pigment goes through different stages of color as it lightens. The amount of change depends on how much pigment the hair has, the strength of the lightening agent, and the length of time it is processed. During the decolorization process, natural hair may go through up to 10 stages of lightening

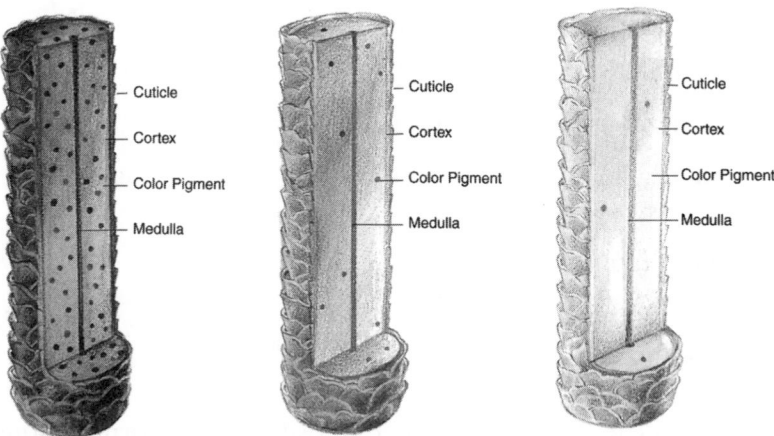

FIGURE 32 | Hair lighteners diffuse pigment.

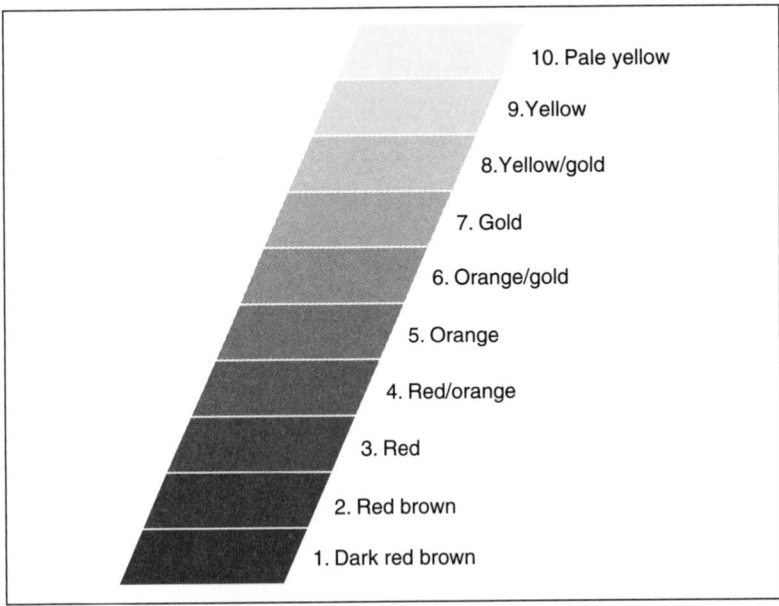

FIGURE 33 | Ten degrees of decolorization.

from the darkest to the lightest. For example, natural black hair can lighten through the brown and/or red stages to orange, gold, to yellow, and finally to pale yellow (Figure 33).

Hair lighteners are used to create blond shades that are not possible with permanent haircolor and to achieve the following:

- lighten the hair to the final shade
- prelightening to prepare the hair for the application of a toner or tint (double-process application)
- lighten hair to a particular shade
- brighten and lighten an existing shade of color

Types of Lighteners

Lighteners are available in three forms: oil, cream, and powder. Oil and cream lighteners are considered *on-the-scalp lighteners* and powder lighteners are *off-the-scalp lighteners*. Each type has unique abilities, chemical compositions, and formulation procedures.

- *Oil lighteners* are usually mixtures of hydrogen peroxide with sulfonated oil. As on-the-scalp lighteners, they are the mildest form of lightener and may be used when only one or two levels of lift are desired.

- *Color oil lighteners* add temporary color and highlight the hair as they lighten. They contain certified colors, may be used without a patch test, and remove pigment while adding color tones. Color oil lighteners are classified according to their action on the hair as follows:

  - Gold: lightens and adds golden to reddish tones depending on the base color of the hair.

  - Silver: lightens and adds silvery highlights to gray or white hair and minimizes red and gold tones in other shades.

  - Red: lightens and adds red highlights.

  - Drab: lightens and adds ash highlights. Tones down or reduces red and gold tones.

  Neutral oil lighteners remove pigment without adding color tone. These oil lighteners may be used to presoften hair for a tint application.

- *Cream lighteners* are the most popular type of on-the-scalp lightener. They contain conditioning agents, bluing, and thickeners, which makes them easy to apply, and will not run, drip, or dry out. Cream lighteners provide the following benefits:

- The conditioning agents give some protection to the hair.

- The bluing agent helps to drab undesirable red and gold tones.

- The thickener provides control during application and prevents overlap.

■ TECH TERM

Sulfonated oil is an organic substance prepared by reacting oils with sulphuric acid. It is used as a base in soapless shampoos and as an emulsifier in hair sprays.

■ *Powder lighteners,* also called paste or quick lighteners, contain an oxygen-releasing booster and inert substances for quicker and stronger action. Paste lighteners will hold and not run, but will dry out quickly and do not contain conditioning agents.

NOTE: If the scalp shows any sensitivity or abrasions, lighteners are not recommended.

Contribution of Underlying Pigment

The natural pigment that remains in the hair after lightening contributes to the artificial color that is added. It is essential to lighten the hair to the correct stage because the pigment that remains in the hair will impact the final result of the hair lightening and coloring process.

Use Figure 34 as a guide to determine the contributing pigment or undertones of color at various hair color levels.

Toners

A toner is a haircoloring product that is applied to prelightened hair for the purpose of achieving the desired color or

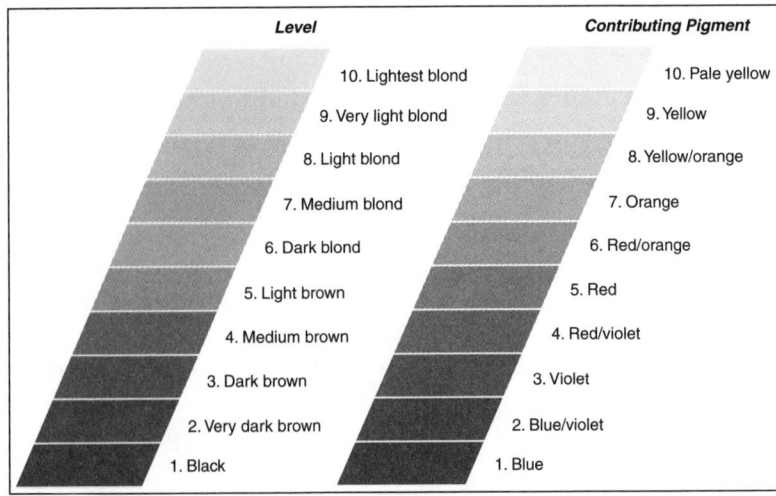

FIGURE 34 | Contributing pigment (undertones).

tones in the hair. Traditional toners are permanent aniline derivative haircoloring products that have a smaller percentage of the formula that creates delicate shades of color. Toners differ from tints only in the degree of color saturation and require a patch test.

Toners are available in pale and delicate colors. They usually have a very different color than the final shade that they produce and may appear to be purple, blue, orange, or pink in the bottle. As toner color oxidizes it goes through several visual color changes; therefore, a strand test should be done to determine the processing time required for a desired shade.

After the hair goes through the desired stages of lightening, the color left in the hair is known as its foundation or contributing color. Achieving the correct foundation is necessary for proper toner development. This is usually the lightest degree of contributing pigment that remains after the lightening process.

Toner manufacturers provide literature that recommends the proper foundation to achieve a desired color. As a general rule, the more pale the desired color, the lighter the foundation must be. It is important to follow the guide closely. Overlightened hair will grab the base color of the toner, while underlightened hair will appear to have more red, yellow, or orange than the intended color.

Because toning is more of a technique than a particular product, semipermanent, demipermanent, and permanent haircolor can also be used as "toners" to achieve the desired hair color.

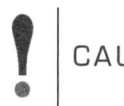

CAUTION

Advise clients that lightening dark hair to a pale blond tone can be very damaging to the hair.

Dye Removers

The removal of haircoloring agents is sometimes desired if the client wants to change to a lighter shade, if a coloring mistake has been made, or if the hair has processed too dark due to an overly porous condition. Dye removers are also known as color or tint removers.

Two basic types of products are available for removing artificial pigment from the hair: an oil-base product, which removes color buildup or stain that is in the cuticle layer of the hair shaft; and a dye solvent, which diffuses and dissolves artificial pigment within the cortical layer.

- *Oil-base dye removers* lift trapped color pigments from cuticle layers and do not create structural changes in the hair shaft or pigment (natural or artificial) of the hair. These dye removers will not make drastic changes in the level of color.

- Dye solvents produce strong lightening effects on melanin and artificial pigment, are nonallergenic, and do not require a predisposition test. Follow manufacturer's directions carefully.

Fillers

Fillers are preparations designed to help equalize excessive porosity and/or to create a color base in the hair. The two general classifications of conditioner fillers are protein and nonprotein, both of which are manufactured in gel, cream, and liquid forms. Color fillers are available in clear, neutral, and a variety of color bases.

Stain Removers

Generally, soap and water will remove most tint stains from the skin. Stain removers are commercially prepared solutions that are designed for this purpose. When soap and water is not capable of removing haircolor from the skin, use one of the following methods:

- Dampen a piece of cotton with the leftover tint. Use a rotary movement to cover the stained areas and follow with a damp towel. Apply a small amount of face cream and wipe clean.

- Use a prepared stain remover.

HAIRCOLORING PROCEDURES TERMINOLOGY

Successful haircoloring usually requires a series of steps to accomplish the desired end result. Due to the wide range of haircoloring products, application methods, and procedures, it is important to have a clear understanding of the terms used in haircoloring processes. Some common procedural terms are *patch test, strand test, soap cap, tint back, record keeping,* and the *client consultation.*

Patch Test

An individual's reaction to aniline derivative tints can be unpredictable. Some clients may show an immediate sensitivity while others may suddenly develop an allergy to the product after years of use. To identify a client who has a sensitivity to aniline derivatives, the U.S. Federal Food, Drug, and Cosmetic Act prescribes that a patch test, also known as a predisposition test, be given 24 to 48 hours prior to each application of an aniline derivative tint or toner.

▷ procedure no. 8

Patch Test

The procedure for performing a patch test is as follows:

1. Select the test area, either behind the ear extending partly into the hairline or on the inside of the elbow.

2. Cleanse an area about the size of a quarter with mild soap and water (Figure 35).

3. Dry the test area by patting with absorbent cotton or a clean towel.

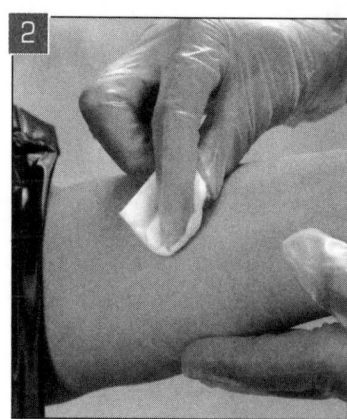

FIGURE 35 | Cleanse the area with mild soap and water.

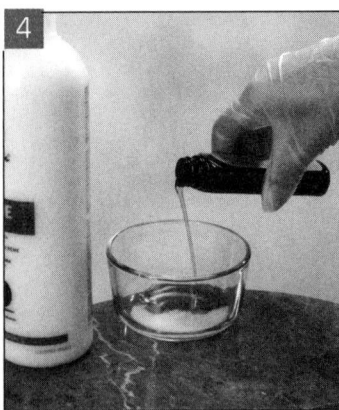

FIGURE 36 | Prepare test solution according to manufacturer's directions.

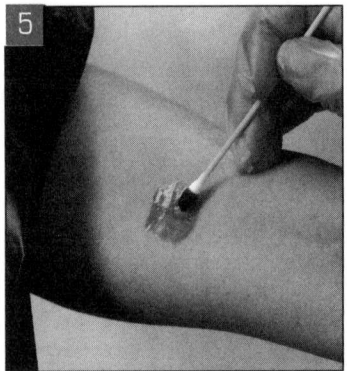

FIGURE 37 | Apply solution to test area.

4 Prepare a small amount of the test solution according to the manufacturer's directions (Figure 36).

5 Apply solution to the test area with a cotton-tipped applicator (Figure 37).

6 Leave the test area uncovered and undisturbed for 24 hours.

7 Examine the test area for either negative or positive reactions.

- A *negative skin test* will show no signs of inflammation and indicates that the color may be safely applied.

- A *positive skin test* is recognized by the presence of redness, swelling, burning, itching, blisters, or eruptions. The client may also suffer from a headache and vomiting. A client showing such symptoms is allergic to aniline derivative tint, and under no circumstances should this particular kind of tint be used. The client should get immediate medical attention to avoid further complications.

8 Record the results on the client record card.

Strand Test

A strand test is performed for color applications to determine how the hair will react to the haircolor product, how long it will take to process, and what the final outcome will look like. After the results of the patch test, the strand test is the next step in performing a haircolor service.

|▷ procedure no. 9

Strand Test

Following the client consultation, scalp and hair analysis, and draping:

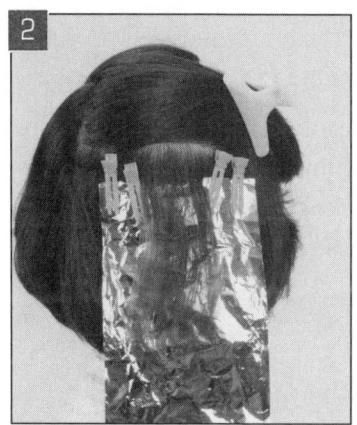

FIGURE 38 | Place the test strand over foil.

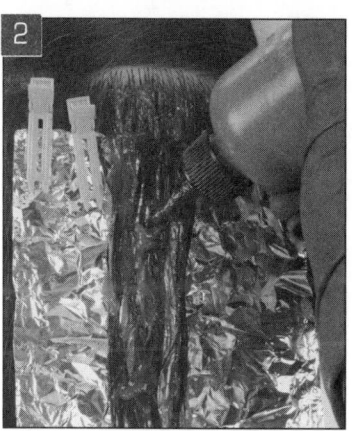

FIGURE 39 | Apply tint to strand.

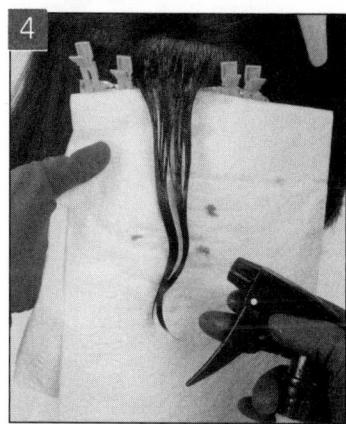

FIGURE 40 | Check strand.

1 Part off a 1/2-inch square parting from the lower crown area just above the occipital. Use plastic clips to secure surrounding hair out of the way.

2 Place the parting of hair over a piece of foil or plastic wrap (Figure 38). Formulate haircolor mixture according to manufacturer's directions and apply to the hair strand (Figure 39).

3 Check the development time at five-minute intervals until the desired color is achieved. Note the time on the record card.

4 Once the color has developed, remove the foil or plastic and place a towel under the section. Mist thoroughly with water, add shampoo, and massage through the strand. Rinse by further misting, towel dry the strand, and observe the results (Figure 40).

5 Adjust the timing, product formulation, or application method as necessary and proceed with the color service.

Soap Cap

A soap cap is a combination of equal parts of a prepared hair-color product and shampoo that is applied like a regular shampoo. Soap caps can be used to brighten existing color, reduce unwanted yellow tones in gray hair, or blend lines of demarcation when a retouch application does not quite match the former color application.

Tint Back

Tint back is the term used to describe the process of returning hair to its natural shade. It is important to keep in mind that previously processed hair will be more porous and, therefore, will process more quickly and possibly darker than intended. In some cases, a filler is required to even out the hair's porosity level or to achieve accurate color correction. A demipermanent haircoloring product is usually an effective choice because it is a deposit-only color formulation with minimal oxidation.

Record Keeping

Before performing a haircoloring service, a client record card should be completed for each client (Figure 41). The client record card is used to log all information pertaining to the haircoloring service. In addition to the client's contact information, the record card should be descriptive enough that it provides preservice and postservice data about the client's hair. For example, key information items should include characteristics of the hair's condition, scalp condition, haircolor history, any corrective treatments, and the results of the haircoloring process. This information can be used for future visits as a basis for other services and should be maintained from one visit to the next.

A release statement form should be used when the client's hair is in a questionable condition that may not withstand chemical processes and treatments. See Figure 42 for a sample barber school release form. To some degree, the release statement is

HAIRCOLOR RECORD

Name _____ Tel. _____

Address _____ City _____

Patch Test: ☐ Negative ☐ Positive   Date _____

Eye Color _____ Skin Tone _____

DESCRIPTION OF HAIR

Form	Length	Texture	Density	Porosity	
☐ straight	☐ short	☐ coarse	☐ sparse	☐ very porous	☐ resistant
☐ wavy	☐ medium	☐ medium	☐ moderate	☐ porous	☐ very resistant
☐ curly	☐ long	☐ fine	☐ thick	☐ normal	☐ perm. waved

Natural hair color _____

	level (1-10)	Tone (Warm, Cool, etc.)	Intensity (Mild, Medium, Strong)

Scalp Condition
☐ normal   ☐ dry   ☐ oily   ☐ sensitive

Condition
☐ normal   ☐ dry   ☐ oily   ☐ faded   ☐ streaked (uneven)

% unpigmented _____ Distribution of unpigmented _____

Previously lightened with _____ for _____ (time)

Previously tinted with _____ for _____ (time)

☐ original hair sample enclosed   ☐ original hair sample not enclosed

Desired hair color _____

	level (1-10)	Tone (Warm, Cool, etc.)	Intensity (Mild, Medium, Strong)

CORRECTIVE TREATMENTS

Color filler used _____ Conditioning treatments with _____

HAIR TINTING PROCESS

whole head _____ retouch inches (cm) _____ shade desired _____

formula: (color/lightener) _____ application technique _____

Results: ☐ good   ☐ poor   ☐ too light   ☐ too dark   ☐ streaked

Comments: _____

_____

_____

_____

_____

Date:	Operator	Price	Date:	Operator	Price

FIGURE 41 | Haircolor record card.

RELEASE FORM

I, the undersigned,_____
                                    (name)

residing at _____
                            (street, address)

_____
                          (city, state and zip)

about to receive chemical services in the

_____

and having been advised that the services shall be performed by either students, graduate students, and/or instructors of the school, in consideration of the nominal charge for such services, hereby release the school, its students, graduate students, instructors, agents, representatives, and/or employees, from any and all claims arising out of and in any way connected with the performance of these services.

The Proprietor Is Not Responsible for Personal Property

Signed _____

Date_____

Witnessed_____

THIS RELEASE FORM MUST BE SIGNED BY THE PARENT OR GUARDIAN IF THE CLIENT BEING SERVED IS UNDER 18 YEARS OF AGE.

FIGURE 42 | Sample school release form.

designed to protect the shop owner from responsibility for accidents and damages and is a requirement of most malpractice insurance. It should be noted, however, that a release statement is not a legally binding contract and will not fully protect the barber or the shop from liability.

Client Consultation

A thorough client consultation is the first step in a haircoloring service (Figure 43). Consultations should be held in a well-lit room that provides either a strong natural light or incandescent

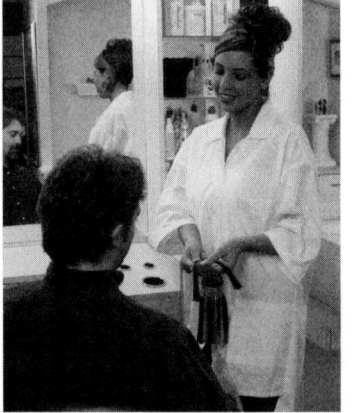

FIGURE 43 | A client consultation should precede every haircolor service.

lighting. Fluorescent lighting is not suitable for judging existing hair colors.

▷ procedure no. 10

Haircoloring Service Consultation

Use the following as a guide to perform a haircoloring service consultation:

1. Drape the client.

2. Have the client fill out a client record card.

3. Perform a hair and scalp analysis and log the results on a record card. Use color swatches to determine client's natural level.

4. Ask the client leading questions about the desired end result, which tells you whether he or she wants temporary or permanent change, all-over color or highlights, and so on.

5. Show examples of appropriate colors and make a determination with the client.

6. Review the procedure, application technique, maintenance, and cost with the client.

7. Gain approval and begin the service.

8. Record end results on the client record card.

■ HAIRCOLOR APPLICATION TERMS

A variety of different haircolor application methods exists. Review the following to become familiar with the terms used in haircoloring procedures.

FOCUS ON

Color Selection

Consider that skin tones change with age. The natural color of the client's hair, which harmonized with the skin coloring at the age of 20 or 30, may seem harsh and unbecoming at the age of 40 or 50. For clients in this age group, keep to the lighter shades of color.

Virgin Application

A *virgin application* refers to the application of haircolor to hair that has not been previously colored. Hair that is in a "virgin" state is usually healthy hair that has not suffered any chemical damage. A virgin application also indicates that the haircoloring product will be applied to the entire hair strand versus the new growth only.

Retouch Application

When permanent haircolor or lighteners are used, new hair growth will become obvious between haircolor applications. The new growth, or regrowth, is that section of the hair shaft between the scalp and the hair that has been previously treated. This creates a line of demarcation between the natural color of the hair and the previously colored or lightened hair that requires blending by way of another color or lightener application. The term *retouch application* is used to describe this blending process.

Single-Process Haircoloring

Single-process haircoloring is a process that lightens and colors the hair in a single application. Examples of single-process coloring are virgin tint applications and tint retouch applications. Single-process haircoloring is also known as single-application coloring, one-step coloring, one-step tinting, and single-application tinting.

Double-Process Haircoloring

Double-process coloring requires two separate and distinct applications to achieve the desired color. The hair is lightened before the depositing color is applied, allowing the practitioner to independently control the lightening and coloring actions. Double-process haircoloring is also known as double-application coloring, two-step coloring, two-step tinting, and double-application tinting. Double-process haircoloring may include the use of lighteners and toners, presofteners and tints, or fillers and color.

Presoftening

Presoftening is the process of treating gray or other extremely resistant hair types to facilitate better color penetration. Presoftening swells and opens the cuticle. It can be accomplished with a mixture of 1 ounce of 20-volume peroxide and 8 drops of 28 percent ammonia water, or with an oil or cream bleach product.

Highlighting

Highlighting is the process of coloring some of the hair strands lighter than the natural or artificial color to add the illusion of sheen and depth. Frosting, tipping, and streaking are forms of highlighting.

Lowlighting

Lowlighting or reverse highlighting is the process of coloring strands or sections of the hair darker than the natural or artificial color. Contrasting dark areas appear to recede and make detail less visible to the eye.

Cap Technique

The *cap technique* involves pulling strands of hair through the holes of a perforated cap with a plastic or metal hook. The number of strands pulled through the cap determines the degree of highlighting or lowlighting that is achieved.

Foil Technique

The *foil technique* involves slicing or weaving out sections of hair to be placed on a piece of foil. The color or lightening product is usually brushed onto the hair section, after which the foil is folded and sealed for processing.

Free-Form Technique

The *free-form technique,* also called *balayage,* is the process of painting a lightener or color directly onto clean, styled hair. The effects can be subtle or dramatic, depending on the type of product (color or lightener) and the amount of hair that it is applied to.

 ## HAIRCOLORING PRODUCT APPLICATIONS

Given the many choices in haircoloring formulations and applications, it is crucial that the barber provides the client with the appropriate product and follows the correct application methods. Use the following as a guide for haircoloring product selection and application.

Temporary Color Rinses

Temporary color rinses may be used to give clients a preview of how a color change will look. They are also a satisfactory option for clients who want to highlight the color of their hair or add slight color to gray hair. These rinses wash out when shampooed and are available in a variety of color shades. Temporary rinses are easily and quickly applied at the shampoo bowl and can serve as an introduction to other longer-lasting color services.

Temporary color rinses can be used to bring out highlights, temporarily restore faded hair color to its natural shade, neutralize yellow tones in white or gray hair, or tone down overlightened hair. Perform a preliminary strand test to determine proper color selection.

▷ procedure no. 11

Temporary Color Rinse Application

Implements and Materials

- ▢ temporary color product
- ▢ applicator bottle (optional)

- ☐ shampoo cape
- ☐ towels
- ☐ protective gloves
- ☐ shampoo
- ☐ color chart
- ☐ record card
- ☐ timer
- ☐ comb

Preparation

If the client is to receive a haircut, perform the cut prior to the color rinse application.

1. Assemble all necessary supplies.

2. Prepare the client. Protect the clothing with a plastic cape and a towel.

3. Examine the client's scalp and hair.

4. Select the desired shade of color rinse.

5. Perform a strand test.

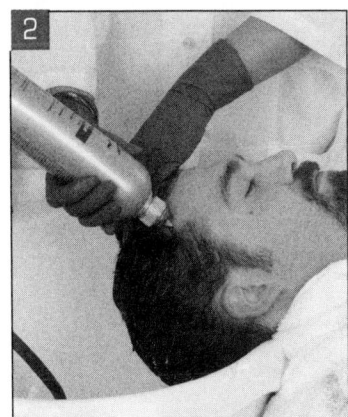

FIGURE 44 │ Apply color rinse at the shampoo bowl.

Procedure

1. Shampoo, rinse, and towel blot hair. Excess moisture must be removed to prevent diluting the color. Put on gloves.

2. With the client reclined at the shampoo bowl, apply the color from the hairline through and around the entire head (Figure 44).

3. Use the comb to blend the color, applying more as necessary for even coverage (Figure 45).

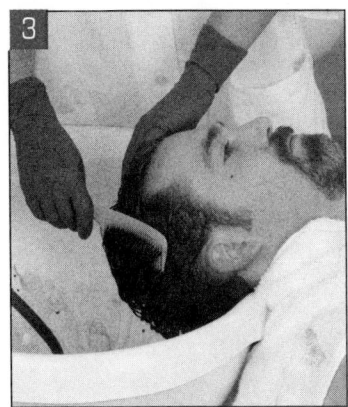

FIGURE 45 │ Blend color rinse through the hair.

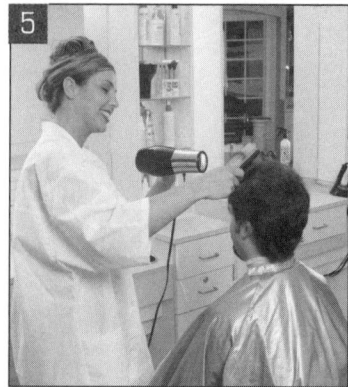

FIGURE 46 | Style the hair.

4   Do not rinse product. Towel blot excess.

5   Proceed with styling (Figure 46).

Cleanup and Sanitation

1   Discard all disposable supplies.

2   Close and wipe off containers and store properly.

3   Sanitize implements, cape, and work area.

4   Wash hands.

5   Record results on client record card.

Semipermanent Haircolor

Semipermanent color products are appropriate for the client who may want more color change than is available with a temporary rinse, but who is hesitant about a permanent color change and its related maintenance. In this way, a semipermanent tint fills the gap between temporary color rinses and permanent haircolor without replacing either of them.

Because semipermanent products are deposit-only colors, the final outcome will depend on the hair's original color and texture, the color that is applied, and the length of development time. These haircoloring products are available in liquid and cream forms in a variety of colors. Some formulations are specifically designed in blue-gray or silver-gray hues to brighten or blend gray color tones.

Characteristics of Semipermanent Tints

The basic characteristics of semipermanent haircolor that influence the decision to choose this color product over another are as follows:

◻ Semipermanent tints do not require the addition of hydrogen peroxide.

- The color is self-penetrating.

- The color is applied the same way each time.

- Retouching is eliminated.

- The color does not rub off, because it has penetrated the hair shaft slightly.

- Hair will usually return to its natural color after four to eight shampoos, provided a mild, nonstripping shampoo is used.

- Semipermanent tints require a 24-hour patch test.

- Some semipermanent haircolors require preshampooing; others do not.

Selecting Semipermanent Color

The addition of artificial color to the natural pigment in the hair shafts creates a darker color. When using a color chart to determine the level and shade of semipermanent color to use, consider the natural color to represent half of the formula. Use the following guide to select the correct color to perform the strand test.

- On hair with no gray (solid), select a color level that is two levels lighter than the desired shade. For example: A client with a natural level of 6 desires a level 7 shade. Therefore, a level 9 shade of color should be used.

- The use of ash or cool shades will create a color that appears darker than if a warm shade is applied.

- Warm colors appear shinier due to the reflection of light.

- For clients with less than 50 percent gray, select a shade that matches the natural hair color.

- For clients with 50 percent or more gray hair, select a color one shade darker than the natural hair color.

▷ procedure no. 12

Semipermanent Color Application

Implements and Materials

- semipermanent color product
- color chart
- applicator bottle or brush
- shampoo cape
- towels
- protective gloves
- shampoo
- conditioner
- comb
- plastic clips (optional, depending on length of hair)
- plastic cap (optional, depending on manufacturer's directions)
- cotton
- protective cream
- record card
- timer

Preparation

1 Perform a preliminary patch test 24 hours before the service. Proceed only if the test is negative.

2 Perform client consultation and record results on client record card.

3 Drape client and apply protective cream.

4 Perform a strand test and record the results.

Procedure

1   Shampoo, rinse, and towel blot hair. Follow manufacturer's directions.

2   Part the hair into four sections. Put on gloves. Apply protective cream to hairline (Figure 47).

3   Working with 1/4-inch to 1/2-inch subsections, apply color to the entire hair shaft from scalp to ends (Figure 48). Use an applicator bottle or brush depending on the product's consistency. With the fingers, gently work the color through the hair until it is thoroughly saturated. Do not massage into the scalp. If the hair is long, pile it loosely on the top of the head.

4   Apply plastic cap if so instructed by the manufacturer's directions.

5   Process according to strand test results and manufacturer's directions. Check color.

6   Following color development, wet client's hair with warm water, lather, and work through hair (Figure 49).

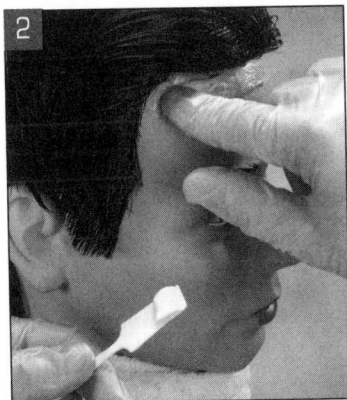

FIGURE 47 │ Apply protective cream around hairline.

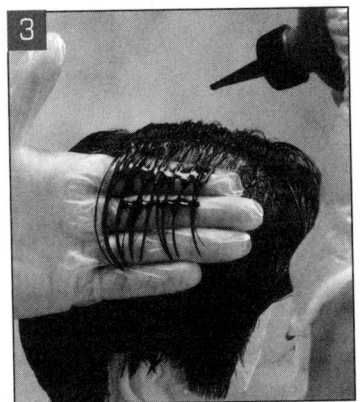

FIGURE 48 │ Apply semipermanent color from scalp to ends.

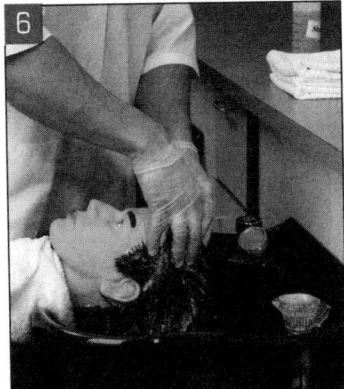

FIGURE 49 │ Work product into a rich lather.

7   Rinse thoroughly, shampoo, and condition. Remove stains as necessary.

8   Rinse, towel blot, and style.

Cleanup and Sanitation

1   Discard all disposable supplies.

2   Close and wipe off containers and store properly.

3   Sanitize implements and tools, cape, and work area.

4   Wash hands.

5   Record results on client record card.

Special Problems

Some semipermanent haircolor products have a tendency to build up on the hair shaft with repeated applications. If this should occur, apply the color to the new growth only, process until the desired color shade develops, then wet the hair with warm water and blend the color through the hair with a large-toothed comb.

Demipermanent Haircolor

Because demipermanent color is considered to be deposit-only color, the same procedures used for the application of a semipermanent haircolor product can be employed. Follow the manufacturer's guidelines for application, color selection, and processing time.

Permanent Haircolor

Practically all professional permanent haircoloring is done with the use of oxidizing penetrating tints that contain aniline derivatives. These penetrating tints are considered either single-process or double-process tints and are available in liquid, cream, and gel forms.

Single-Process Haircoloring

Single-process tints provide a simplified method of haircoloring. In one application, the hair can be colored permanently without requiring preshampooing, presoftening, or prelightening. Single-process tints usually contain a lightening agent, shampoo, aniline derivative tint, and an alkalizing agent to activate the peroxide. Most color is formulated for use with 20-volume hydrogen peroxide. When other volumes of peroxide are used, the color results change. The choice of colors varies from deepest black to lightest blond.

Characteristics of Single-Process Tints

A single-application tint is applied on dry hair. If the hair is extremely oily or dirty and a shampoo is necessary, it must be dried thoroughly before applying the tint. Some characteristics of single-process tints are that they:

- save time by eliminating preshampooing or prelightening.
- color the hair lighter or darker than the client's natural color.
- blend in gray or white hair to match the client's natural hair color.
- tone down streaks, off-shades, discoloration, and faded hair ends.

Color Selection of Single-Process Tints

The porosity of the hair is one of the most important characteristics to consider when choosing hair color tint shades. Use the following guide for choosing the level of color when tinting darker.

- Normal porosity: half level lighter than desired color
- Slightly porous: one level lighter than desired color
- Very porous: one to two levels lighter than desired color

General rules for single-process color selection for gray hair are:

- To match the natural color of hair and to cover gray, select the color closest to the natural shade.
- To brighten or lighten hair color and to cover gray, select a shade lighter than the natural color. The selected tint must contain enough color to produce the desired shade on gray hair.
- To darken the hair and cover gray, select a color darker than the natural hair color.
- Study the manufacturer's color chart for correct color selections.

Use the following formula for color selection when tinting lighter than the natural color.

FORMULATION STEP EXAMPLE:

1. Identify the desired level.   6
2. Identify the natural level.   −4
3. Subtract the natural level from the desired level.   2
4. Add the level difference to the desired level.   +6
5. Total is the level of color needed.   8

▷ procedure no. 13

Single-Process Color Application for Virgin Hair

Implements and Materials

- single-process permanent color product
- hydrogen peroxide

- color chart
- applicator bottle or brush and bowl
- shampoo cape
- towels
- protective gloves
- shampoo
- conditioner
- comb
- plastic clips (optional, depending on length of hair)
- plastic cap (optional, depending on manufacturer's directions)
- cotton
- protective cream
- record card
- timer

Preparation

1. Perform a preliminary patch test 24 hours before the service. Proceed only if the test is negative.

2. Perform client consultation and record results on client record card.

3. Drape client and apply protective cream.

4. Perform a strand test and record the results.

Procedure for Single-Process Permanent Color Application

1. Follow manufacturer's directions.

2. Put on gloves and part dry hair into four sections (Figure 50).

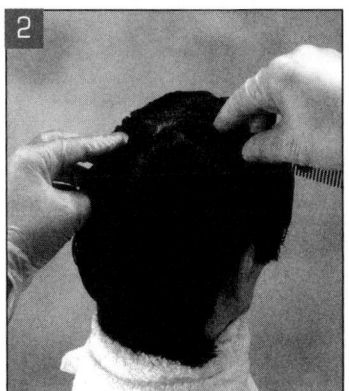

FIGURE 50 | Part hair into four sections.

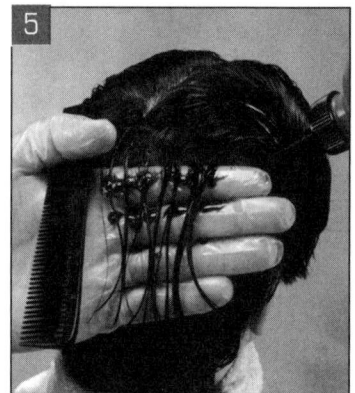

FIGURE 51 | Apply color to midshaft.

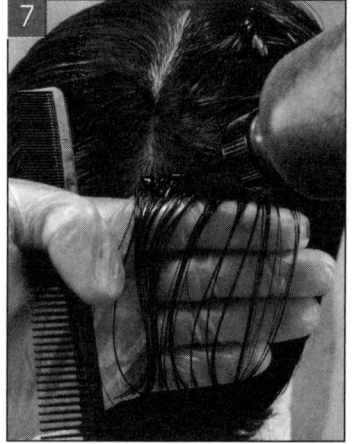

FIGURE 52 | Apply product to scalp area.

3 Prepare color formula for either bottle or brush application method.

4 Begin in the section where the hair is most resistant or where there will be the most color change.

5 Part off 1/4-inch subsections and apply color to the midshaft area (Figure 51). Stay at least 1/2 inch from the scalp and do not apply to the porous ends.

6 Process according to the strand test results and the manufacturer's directions.

7 Check color development. When desired color is reached, apply remaining product to hair at the scalp, then pull the color through to the hair ends (Figures 52 and 53).

8 Lightly wet client's hair with warm water and lather. Massage lather through the hair.

9 Rinse thoroughly, shampoo, and condition. Remove stains as necessary.

10 Rinse, towel blot, and style (Figure 54).

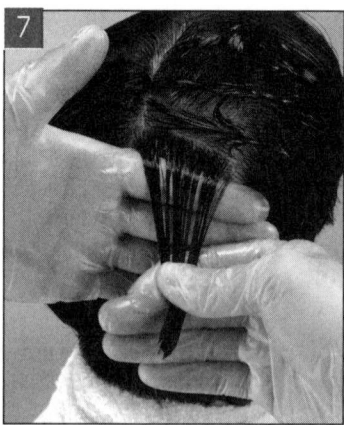

FIGURE 53 | Pull color through to hair ends.

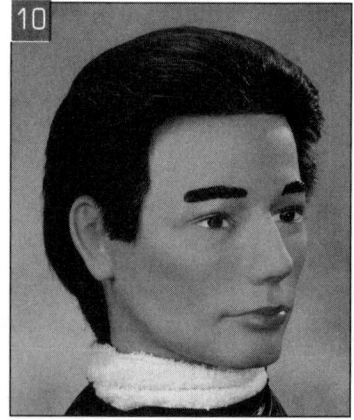

FIGURE 54 | Style as desired by client.

Cleanup and Sanitation

1. Discard all disposable supplies.

2. Close and wipe off containers and store properly.

3. Sanitize implements and tools, cape, and work area.

4. Wash hands.

5. Record results on client record card.

▷ procedure no. 14

Single-Process Color Retouch

To retouch new hair growth, use the same preparation steps as for coloring virgin hair. Then proceed as follows:

1. Refer to the client record card for correct color selection and other data.

2. Apply the tint first to new growth at sideburns, temples, and nape area.

3. Apply the tint to new growth in 1/4-inch strands. Do not overlap. Check frequently for color development.

4. When color has almost developed, dilute the remaining tint by adding a mild shampoo or warm water. Apply and gently work the mixture through the hair with the fingertips. Comb and blend from the scalp to the hair ends for even distribution.

5. Process for the required time. Rinse with warm water to remove excess color.

6. Use an acid-balanced shampoo and rinse thoroughly.

7. Dry and comb, or style hair as desired.

8. Remove color stains, if necessary.

9 Fill out a record card.

10 Clean up in the usual manner.

Double-Process Haircoloring

Double-process haircoloring begins with hair lightening, followed by a tint or toner application. This double process requires two separate steps as presented in the following section.

Characteristics of Lighteners

Lightening creates a desired color foundation. This new color foundation may be the finished result or it may be the first step of a double-process application. Consideration must be given to the existing hair color, processing and development time, resulting porosity, and color selection to achieve the desired shade.

Depending on the manufacturer's directions, hair lighteners can be used for the following processes.

- to lighten the entire head of hair
- to lighten the hair to a particular shade
- to brighten and lighten the existing shade
- to tip, streak, or frost certain sections of the hair
- to lighten hair that has already been tinted
- to remove undesirable casts and off-shades
- to correct dark streaks or spots in hair that has already been lightened or tinted

Selection of Lighteners

Remember to choose the appropriate lightener for the service. Cream and oil lighteners may be used on the scalp; powder lighteners are off-the-scalp products.

Together with the manufacturer's directions, be guided by the following general rules when choosing a lightening product:

- Oil lighteners are the mildest form of lightener and may be used when only one or two levels of lift are desired.

- Cream lighteners offer some protection to the hair, are controllable during application, and can be used to drab undesirable red and gold tones. For increased strength, up to three activators can be added for on-the-scalp applications and up to four activators for off-the-scalp processes.

- Powder lighteners are strong enough to produce blonding effects, but should not be used for retouch applications.

▷ procedure no. 15

Step 1: Lightening Virgin Hair

Implements and Materials

- lightener product
- hydrogen peroxide
- color chart
- applicator bottle or brush and bowl
- shampoo cape
- towels
- protective gloves
- shampoo
- conditioner
- comb

- ☐ plastic clips (optional, depending on length of hair)
- ☐ cotton
- ☐ protective cream
- ☐ record card
- ☐ timer

Preparation

1. Perform a preliminary patch test 24 hours before the service. Proceed only if the test is negative.

2. Perform client consultation and record results on client record card.

3. Drape client and apply protective cream.

4. Perform a strand test and record the results.

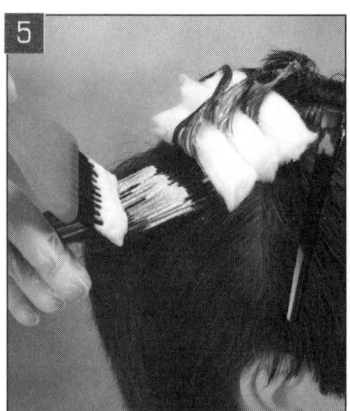

FIGURE 55 | Apply lightener to top and underside of the subsection.

Procedure

1. Divide dry hair into four sections.

2. Apply protective cream around hairline. Put on gloves.

3. Prepare lightening formula. Use either bottle or brush application method.

4. Begin in the section where the hair is most resistant or where there will be the most color change.

5. Part off 1/8-inch subsections and apply lightener 1/2 inch from the scalp up to, but not through, the porous ends. Apply to top and underside of the subsection and place a strip of cotton along the part lines to prevent seepage to the scalp area (Figures 55 and 56).

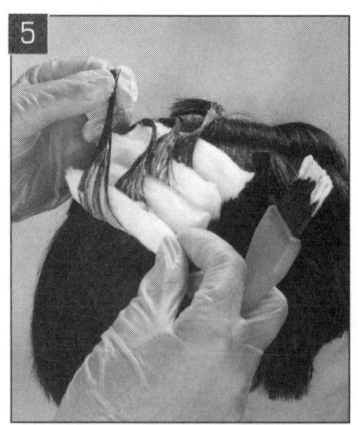

FIGURE 56 | Place a strip of cotton along the part lines.

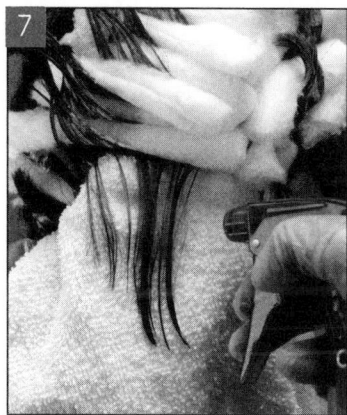

FIGURE 57 | Test for lightening action.

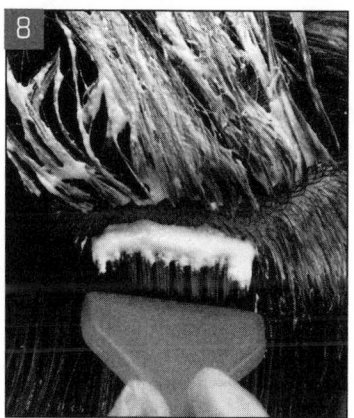

FIGURE 58 | Remove cotton and apply lightener near the scalp.

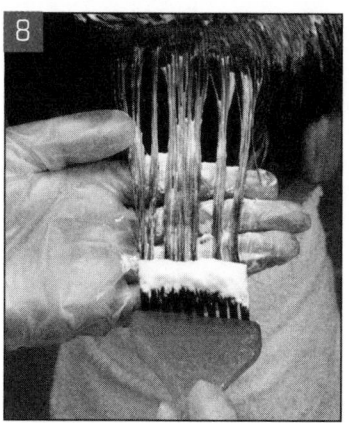

FIGURE 59 | Apply lightening products to the ends.

6   Apply lightener to other sections in the same manner. Keep lightener moist with repeated applications if necessary. Do not comb the lightener through the hair.

7   Process according to the strand test results and manufacturer's directions. Check lightening action by misting as for a strand test about 15 minutes before the completion of the time required (Figure 57). If the level is not light enough, reapply the mixture and continue testing frequently until the desired shade is almost developed.

8   Remove cotton from scalp area and apply lightener near the scalp (Figure 58). Apply lightening product to the porous ends (Figure 59). Process until the entire hair shaft has reached the desired level.

9   Rinse thoroughly, shampoo, and condition. Dry the hair with a towel or under a cool dryer per the manufacturer's directions. Examine the scalp for abrasions.

10 Proceed with toner application if desired.

Cleanup and Sanitation

1. Discard all disposable supplies.

2. Close and wipe off containers and store properly.

3. Sanitize implements and tools, cape, and work area.

4. Wash hands.

5. Record results on client record card.

Lightener Retouch

A *lightener retouch* is the term commonly used when a lightener is applied only to the new hair growth to match the rest of the lightened hair. The client's record card should be consulted as a guide to the lightener used previously and the time required for the shade to develop.

Cream lightener generally is used for a lightener retouch because it prevents the overlapping of the previously lightened hair. Black or dark brown hair usually requires more frequent retouch applications than lighter natural shades. When retouching, the lightener is applied to the new growth only. If a lighter or different level is desired overall, wait until the new growth is almost light enough or has developed fully. Then bring the remainder of the lightener through the hair shaft. One to five minutes should be ample time to create a lighter level effect.

Toners

Other than a reduced ratio of dye load in the formula, toners have the same chemical ingredients and actions as permanent haircolor products. The difference in the formulation is what allows for toners to deliver pale, delicate shades of color to prelightened hair.

Color Selection of Toners

Pastel colors, such as silver, ash, platinum, and beige, are popular toners for lighter blond colors. Gray hair and skin tone changes that accompany advancing years may benefit from the lighter silver tones. When extremely pale toner shades such as very light silver, platinum, or beige are desired, the hair must be prelightened to pale yellow or almost white.

▷ procedure no. 16

Step 2: Toner Application

Implements and Materials

- ◘ toner product
- ◘ hydrogen peroxide
- ◘ color chart
- ◘ applicator bottle or brush and bowl
- ◘ shampoo cape
- ◘ towels
- ◘ protective gloves
- ◘ shampoo
- ◘ conditioner
- ◘ comb
- ◘ plastic clips (optional, depending on length of hair)
- ◘ cotton
- ◘ protective cream
- ◘ record card
- ◘ timer

Preparation

1 Perform a preliminary patch test 24 hours before the service. Proceed only if the test is negative.

2. Perform client consultation and record results on client record card.

3. Drape client.

4. Prelighten the hair to the desired level.

5. Shampoo, rinse, condition, and towel dry the hair.

6. Perform a strand test and record the results.

Procedure

1. Divide dry hair into four sections.

2. Apply protective cream around hairline. Put on gloves.

3. If using an oxidative toner, mix the toner and developer. Use either bottle or brush application method.

4. Begin in the crown section and part off 1/4-inch subsections. Apply toner from the scalp up to, but not through, the porous ends. Apply to other sections.

5. Process according to the strand test results and the manufacturer's directions. Check toning action by misting as for a strand test. If proper color development has occurred, work the toner through the ends of the hair.

6. When the desired color has been reached, add water and massage toner into a lather.

7. Rinse thoroughly, shampoo, and condition. Remove any stains as necessary.

8. Style as desired.

Cleanup and Sanitation

1 Discard all disposable supplies.

2 Close and wipe off containers and store properly.

3 Sanitize implements and tools, cape, and work area.

4 Wash hands.

5 Record results on client record card.

Toner Retouch

A toner retouch must be given the same careful consideration as you would give a two-color tint retouch application. The new growth must be prelightened to the same degree of lightness achieved in the previous toner application. The lightener is applied to the new growth only. To avoid damage to the hair, be careful not to overlap the lightener on previously lightened hair. After the lightening process has been completed, the toner is applied to the entire length of the hair in the usual manner.

Suggestions and Reminders

- Toners are completely dependent on the proper preliminary lightening treatment, which must leave the hair light and porous enough to receive the pale toner shades.

- Semipermanent and demipermanent color can also be used with lighteners to achieve specific tones and colors.

- Strand tests are vital to correct double-process applications.

- A complete explanation of the possible outcome should be discussed with the client. It is always possible that the hair cannot be decolorized sufficiently for the color choice without resulting in serious damage to the hair. Gold or red pigments remaining in the hair after lightening indicate underlightening; ash tones indicate overlightening. When this happens, the shade of toner should be chosen to neutralize the unwanted tones.

SPECIAL-EFFECTS HAIRCOLORING AND LIGHTENING

Special-effects haircoloring refers to any technique that involves the partial lightening or coloring of the hair. As previously defined in the Haircolor Application Terms section, *highlighting* is the process of lightening or coloring some of the hair strands lighter than the natural color. Frosting, tipping, and streaking are forms of highlighting application techniques. *Lowlighting,* or reverse highlighting, is the process of coloring strands or sections of the hair darker than the natural color. As an application process, tipping and streaking techniques can be used for lowlighting effects.

Frosting involves lightening strands of hair over various parts of the head. Either the cap technique or *foils* can be used for the process. The effect achieved will depend on where and how many strands of hair are treated.

Tipping is similar to frosting, except that only the ends of the hair strands are lightened or colored. Apply the product using either the cap technique or free-form technique for better placement and product control.

Streaking is also similar to frosting, but the strands of lightened or colored hair are usually thicker and more dramatic than those taken for a frosting effect. Streaking effects are best accomplished using the foil or free-form application techniques.

Cap Technique

As we have learned, the cap technique involves pulling strands of hair through the holes of a perforated cap with a plastic or metal hook (Figure 60). The number of strands pulled through the cap determines the degree of highlighting or lowlighting that is achieved throughout the hair.

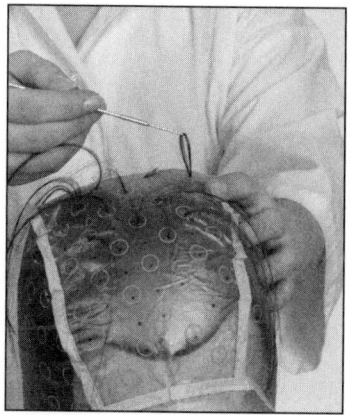

FIGURE 60 | Draw strands through holes in the cap.

▷ procedure no. 17

Cap Technique

1. Perform a preliminary patch test 24 hours before the service. Proceed only if the test is negative.

2. Perform client consultation and record results on client record card.

3. Drape client.

4. Perform a strand test and record the results.

5. Shampoo and dry the hair.

6. Comb the hair gently.

7. Adjust a perforated cap over the head.

8. Draw the strands of hair through the holes with crochet hook. Prepare coloring or lightening product. Put on gloves.

9. Apply the color or lightener.

10. Cover loosely with a plastic cap if necessary for processing.

11. When the hair has processed remove the plastic cap if present.

12. Rinse and shampoo the color or lightener with the perforated cap in place. Towel dry.

13. *Optional:* Apply toner if necessary and process accordingly.

14 Style as desired.

15 Perform cleanup and sanitation procedures.

Foil Technique

The foil technique involves weaving out alternating strands of hair from a subsection, or slicing out 1/8-inch partings from a straight part, to isolate the strands for coloring or lightening. The selected strands are then placed over a piece of foil wrap and the color or lightening product is applied. The foil is folded to prevent coloring or lifting any of the unwoven hair, and strands are processed to the desired shade. The foil technique facilitates strategically placed color or highlights that can accentuate a haircut or style. Frosting and streaking effects can be accomplished using the foil technique.

▷ procedure no. 18

Foil Technique

1 Perform a preliminary patch test 24 hours before the service. Proceed only if the test is negative.

2 Perform client consultation and record results on client record card.

3 Drape client.

4 Perform a strand test and record the results.

5 Apply to dry hair if using permanent color or lighteners. Apply to damp hair if using traditional semipermanent colors.

6 Comb the hair gently. Prepare color or lightening product. Put on gloves.

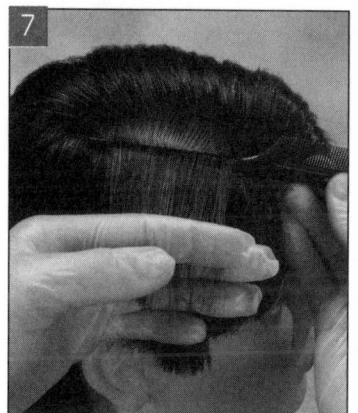

FIGURE 61 | Slicing out the strands.

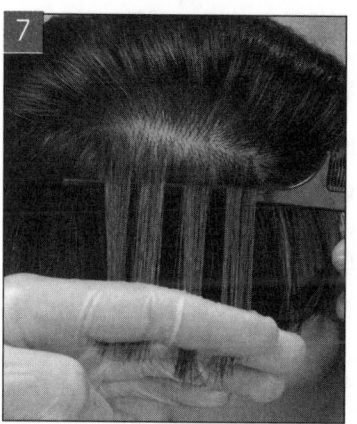

FIGURE 62 | Weaving out the strands.

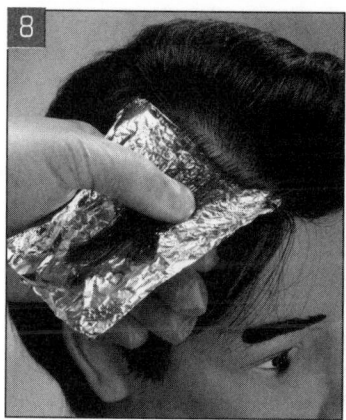

FIGURE 63 | Place foil under hair section.

7 Slice or weave out the strands from the first parting to be processed (Figures 61 and 62).

8 Place the foil under the hair and grasp it firmly at the scalp between the thumb and index finger (Figure 63).

9 Brush color or lightening product onto the hair (Figure 64).

10 Fold the foil in half from bottom to top until the ends meet at the scalp area (Figure 65).

11 Fold the left and right edges of the foil halfway and crimp lightly until secure (Figure 66). Clip the foil upward.

12 Continue the same process until all the areas to be foiled are completed (Figure 67).

13 Process according to strand test results. Check color or lightening level.

14 When processing is complete, remove foils at the shampoo bowl.

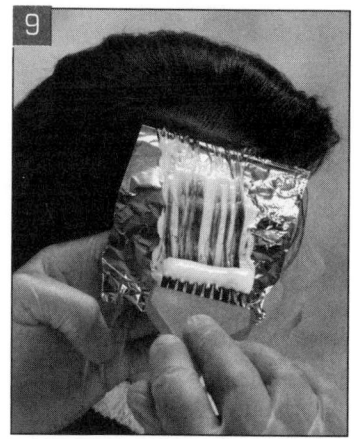

FIGURE 64 | Brush product onto the hair.

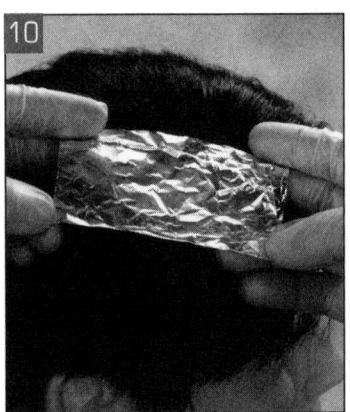

FIGURE 65 │ Fold foil from bottom to top.

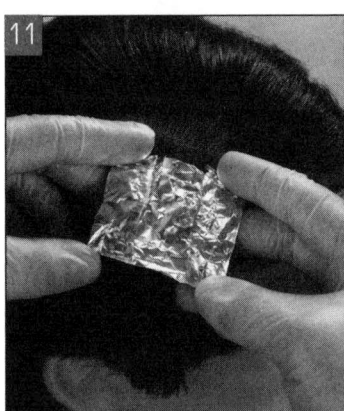

FIGURE 66 │ Fold left and right edges.

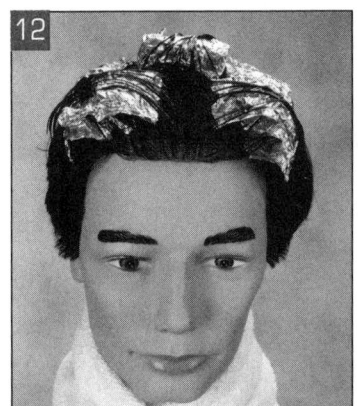

FIGURE 67 │ Completed foil wrap.

15 Rinse, shampoo, and condition according to product directions.

16 Style hair as desired.

17 Perform cleanup and sanitation procedures

Note: When performing the foil technique over the entire head, the sequence of application should be: lower crown, back, sides, top, and front.

SPECIAL PROBLEMS AND CORRECTIVE HAIRCOLOR

Each haircoloring or lightening service has the potential to create unique problems. Some problems can be avoided by performing preliminary strand tests, but others can be the result of unique properties within the client's hair structure that are unforeseen. Most haircoloring and lightening problems can be resolved with a calm approach, an accurate assessment of the problem, and the knowledge to rectify the situation.

Gray Hair Challenges

Gray, white, or salt-and-pepper hair shades have characteristics that can present unique color challenges (Figure 68). Because both gray and white hair contain little melanin within the cortex, a large number of coloring services are performed with the intent to cover or enhance the color. Depending on the amount of gray, the hair may have a yellowish cast or process differently from one strand to another. Some gray hair also tends to be more resistant to chemical processes and may require presoftening before a service.

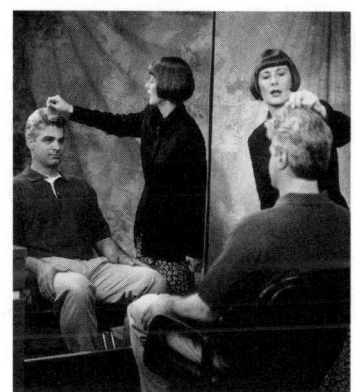

FIGURE 68 | Gray hair presents certain challenges.

Yellowed Hair

Gray, white, and salt-and-pepper hair with a yellowish cast can be treated with violet-based colors that range from highlighting shampoos and temporary rinses to lightening agents. The longevity of the product used will depend on the client's desired result and the options offered by the barber. (If lightening and coloring services are not typically offered in the barbershop, it is highly recommended that, at a minimum, highlighting shampoos or temporary rinses with violet bases be available to shop clients.)

Determining the Percentage of Gray

Because most people retain some dark hair as they turn gray, the hair must be analyzed for level, hue, and the percentage of gray before the appropriate product selection can be made. Gray hair may be evenly distributed or isolated in various sections of the head, such as the temple areas. Use Table 5 as a guide for determining percentages of gray and recommended formulations.

Formulating for Gray Hair

Gray hair will usually accept the level of the color applied. Generally, lighter shades in the level-9 range may not provide complete coverage, whereas levels 6, 7, and 8 will often cover successfully. The difference in coverage ability is due to the

Table 5	PERCENTAGES OF GRAY AND RECOMMENDED FORMULATIONS		
PERCENTAGE OF GRAY	**CHARACTERISTICS**	**SEMIPERMANENT COLOR FORMULATION**	**PERMANENT COLOR FORMULATION**
90–100%	Virtually no pigment; white	Desired level	Desired level
70–90%	Mostly nonpigmented	Equal parts: desired level & one level lighter	Two parts desired level & one part lighter level
50–70%	More gray and pigmented	One level lighter than desired level	Equal parts: desired level & lighter level
30–50%	More pigmented than gray	Equal parts: one level lighter & two levels lighter	Two parts lighter level & one part desired level
10–30%	Mostly pigmented	Two levels lighter than desired color	One level lighter

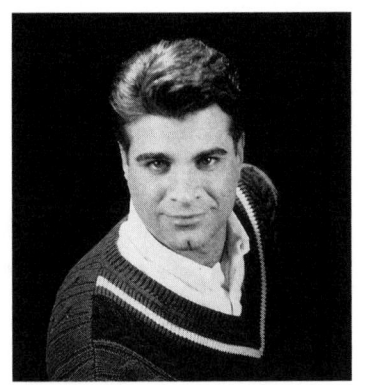

FIGURE 69 | Many haircolor options cover gray successfully.

smaller percentage of artificial pigments found in the lighter shades of a level-9 formulation.

When a client has 80–100 percent gray, lighter haircolors are usually more flattering than darker shades. The client's skin tone, eye color, and personal preference will determine whether warm or cool tones are used. Reminder: When a dark level of color is applied to hair with a low percentage of gray, the addition of artificial pigment to the natural pigment will create a color that may be darker than the intended result. In addition, the nonpigmented strands may process lighter. To avoid these outcomes, select a color that is one level lighter than the darkest natural color (Figure 69).

Occasionally, gray hair is so resistant that presoftening is necessary for better color penetration. Mix the product according to the manufacturer's directions and apply to the most resistant areas first. Process as directed and then perform a preliminary strand test with the desired color.

Fillers

Color fillers are dual-purpose haircoloring products that are able to create a color base and equalize excessive porosity in one application.

They are available in clear, neutral, and a variety of colors. A clear filler is designed to correct porosity without affecting color and does not deposit a color base. Neutral fillers (a balance of all three primary colors) have minimal saturation and color correction abilities but have full power to equalize porosity. Color fillers are preoxidized colors that remain true during application and that will be subdued by the tint.

If there is any doubt that the finished color will develop into an even shade, a color filler is recommended. The filler is applied after the hair has been prelightened and before the application of a toner or tint. Fillers are also used for clients who have tinted or lightened hair and desire to return it to the natural color. Color fillers have the ability to:

- deposit color to faded hair shafts and ends.
- help hair to hold color.
- help to ensure a uniform color from the scalp to the hair ends.
- prevent color streaking.
- prevent off-color results.
- prevent dullness.
- facilitate more uniform color in a tint back to the natural shade.

Fillers use certified colors as pigments and are safe to use without a predisposition test. They may be used directly from the container and applied to the hair prior to tinting, or may be added to the remainder of the tint and applied to damaged hair ends. To obtain satisfactory results, select the color filler to match the same basic shade as the toner or tint to be used.

Reconditioning Damaged Hair

Hair that is damaged due to careless chemical applications, excessive heat, or misused styling products must be reconditioned before it can be tinted or lightened successfully.

Hair may need reconditioning for reasons other than damage resulting from the use of harmful products. Sometimes hair is naturally brittle, thin, and lifeless. Both neglect and the client's physical condition may contribute to these conditions.

Hair is considered damaged when it exhibits one or more of the following characteristics:

- overporous condition
- brittle and dry
- breaks easily
- little to no elasticity
- rough and harsh to the touch
- spongy and mats easily when wet
- rejects color or absorbs too much color during a tinting process

Any of these conditions may create undesirable results during a tinting or lightening treatment. Therefore, damaged hair should receive reconditioning treatments prior to and after the application of these chemical agents.

Reconditioning Treatment

To restore damaged hair to a more normal condition, commercial products containing lanolin or protein substances should be used. The reconditioning agent is applied for 10–20 minutes and rinsed from the hair. If heat is applied, use a heating cap, a steamer, or a heating lamp according to the manufacturer's directions.

Tint Back to Natural Color

Clients who have been tinting or lightening their hair may want to return to their natural shade. Each tint back to natural color must be handled as an individual situation. The determining factors in the selection of the tint shade are the present condition and color of the hair, the final result desired, and the original color. Check the natural shade of the hair next to the scalp.

Select an appropriate shade of filler to correspond with the tint to be used; otherwise it will be difficult to obtain a uniform color from the scalp to hair ends, due to uneven porosity levels. Perform strand tests as needed to determine the expected final outcome.

Coating Dyes

Many clients buy and use over-the-counter haircoloring products at home. Some such coloring agents are actually progressive dyes and must be removed prior to any other chemical service.

Hair treated with a compound, metallic, or other coating dye looks dry and dull and generally feels harsh and brittle to the touch. These colors usually fade to unnatural tones. Silver dyes have a greenish cast, lead dyes leave a purple color, and those containing copper turn red. If the barber is unsure as to whether the client has used a progressive dye, a test for metallic salts and dyes should be performed on the hair.

▷ procedure no. 19

Test for Metallic Salts and Coating Dyes

1. In a glass container, mix 1 ounce (30 ml) of 20-volume (6 percent) peroxide and 20 drops of 28 percent ammonia water.

2 Cut a few strands of the client's hair, bind it with tape, and immerse it in the solution for 30 minutes.

3 Remove, towel dry, and observe the strand. Refer to the following for analysis of the hair:

- Hair dyed with lead will lighten immediately.

- Hair treated with silver will show no reaction at all. This indicates that other chemicals will not be successful because they will not be able to penetrate the coating.

- Hair treated with copper will start to boil, and will pull apart easily. This hair would be severely damaged or destroyed if other chemicals such as those found in permanent colors or perm solutions were applied to it.

- Hair treated with a coating dye either will not change color or will lighten in spots. Hair in this condition will not receive chemical services easily and the length of time necessary for penetration may result in further damage to the hair.

▷ procedure no. 20

Removing Coatings from the Hair

The removal of metallic dyes from the hair shaft may not always be effective the first time. Performing a strand test after the treatment will indicate whether the metallic deposits have been removed. If not, the entire application must be repeated until the hair shaft is sufficiently free of metal salts to perform other chemical services.

Materials Needed

- ◘ 70 percent alcohol
- ◘ concentrated shampoo for oily hair

◘ mineral, castor, vegetable, or commercially prepared color-removing oil

Procedure

1   Apply 70 percent alcohol to dry hair.

2   Allow alcohol to stand for five minutes.

3   Apply the oil to the hair thoroughly.

4   Cover the hair completely with a plastic cap.

5   Place under a hot dryer for 30 minutes.

6   To remove, saturate with concentrated shampoo.

7   Work the shampoo into the oil for three minutes, then rinse with warm water.

8   Repeat the shampoo steps until the oil is removed completely.

COLORING MUSTACHES AND BEARDS

An aniline derivative tint should never be used for coloring mustaches; to do so may cause serious irritation or damage to the lips or the delicate membranes of the nostrils. Harmless commercial products are available in a variety of formulations that are appropriate for coloring mustaches and beards.

Crayons are waxy sticks that are available in several colors: blond, medium and dark brown, black, and auburn. The end of the stick is used like a pencil to apply the product by rubbing it directly on the facial hair until the desired shade is reached.

Pomades usually consist of harmless ingredients and are formulated specifically for coloring mustaches and beards. These products are available in a variety of shades including black, brown, blond, chestnut, and white (neutral). The pomade is applied to the facial hair with a small brush and is stroked from the nostrils downward until full coverage is achieved.

Liquid pomades are also available and may be preferred for use on beards. Some pomades contain heavy waxing ingredients that can be used to style mustaches with rolled or twisted ends for dramatic looks. Liquid eyebrow and eyelash tint is also available in brown and black for coloring facial hair.

▷ procedure no. 21

Coloring Mustaches and Beards

Implements and Materials

- petroleum jelly
- coloring solutions (No. 1 and No. 2)
- stain remover
- towels
- applicator sticks

Procedure

1. Seat the client in a comfortable position and drape.

2. Place a clean towel across the chest.

3. Wash the facial hair with warm, soapy water.

4. Apply petroleum jelly around the hairline of the facial hair.

5. Apply solution No. 1. Remove the cap and moisten a cotton-tipped applicator in the solution. Touch the tip of the applicator to a towel to remove excess moisture. Apply the solution to the mustache/beard, moistening it completely. Replace the cap on bottle

No. 1. Discard the applicator immediately. Moisten a fresh cotton-tipped applicator with stain remover and place it on the edge of a towel for future use. Replace the cap on the stain remover bottle.

6. Apply solution No. 2 to the mustache/beard in the same manner as solution No. 1. If the skin becomes stained, use stain remover immediately. Replace the cap on bottle No. 2.

7. Wash the mustache/beard with soap and cool water.

8. Remove any stains with stain remover. Replace the bottle cap.

9. Style the mustache/beard as desired.

10. Clean up in the usual manner.

HAIRCOLORING SAFETY PRECAUTIONS

- Perform a 24-hour patch test before the application of a tint or toner.
- Examine the scalp before applying a tint.
- Do not apply tint if abrasions are present on the scalp.
- Use only sanitized swabs, brushes, applicator bottles, combs, and linens.
- Always wash your hands before and after serving a client.
- Do not brush the hair prior to a tint.
- Do not apply permanent haircolor immediately following a permanent wave.
- Do not apply a tint without reading the manufacturer's directions.
- Perform a strand test for color and processing results.

- ☐ Choose a shade of tint that harmonizes with the general complexion.
- ☐ Use an applicator bottle or bowl (plastic or glass) for mixing the tint.
- ☐ Do not mix tint long before its use; discard leftover tint.
- ☐ If required, use the correct shade of color filler.
- ☐ Perform frequent strand tests until the desired shade is reached.
- ☐ Suggest a reconditioning treatment for tinted hair.
- ☐ Do not apply tint if metallic or compound dye is present.
- ☐ Do not apply tint if a patch test is positive.
- ☐ Give a strand test for the correct color shade before applying tint.
- ☐ Do not use an alkaline or harsh shampoo for tint removal.
- ☐ Do not use water that is too hot for removing tint.
- ☐ Protect the client's clothing by proper draping.
- ☐ Do not permit tint to come in contact with the client's eyes.
- ☐ Do not overlap during a tint retouch.
- ☐ Do not neglect to fill out a tint record card.
- ☐ Do not apply hydrogen peroxide or any material containing hydrogen peroxide directly over dyes known or believed to contain a metallic salt. Breakage or complete disintegration of the hair may result.
- ☐ Wear protective gloves.

HAIR LIGHTENING SAFETY PRECAUTIONS

▢ Analyze the condition of the hair and suggest reconditioning treatments, if required.

▢ When working with a cream or paste lightener, it must be the thickness of whipped cream to avoid dripping or running, causing overlapping.

▢ Apply lightener to resistant areas first. Pick up 1/8-inch sections when applying lightener. This will ensure complete coverage.

▢ Check strands frequently until the desired shade is reached.

▢ After completing the lightener application, check the skin and remove any lightener from these areas.

▢ Check the towel around the client's neck. Lightener on the towel that is allowed to come in contact with the skin will cause irritation.

▢ Lightened hair is fragile and requires special care. Use only a very mild shampoo, and cool water for rinsing.

▢ If a preliminary shampoo is necessary, comb the hair carefully. Avoid irritating the scalp during the shampoo or when combing the hair.

▢ Work as rapidly as possible when applying the lightener to produce a uniform shade without streaking.

▢ Never allow lightener to stand; use it immediately.

▢ Cap all bottles to avoid loss of strength.

▢ Keep a completed record card of all lightening treatments.

reminder

Keep up-to-date—manufacturers are constantly improving and developing new haircoloring products. Be sure to attend seminars and trade shows as often as possible to stay current in your profession.

FINAL THOUGHTS

In the preceding sections, we covered the basics of nonsurgical hair restoration and hair coloring services—two service areas that can dramatically impact your clients' personal appearance. By offering these services, you will be in a position to meet the needs of the growing number of men who are looking to their barber or stylist to provide them with a subtle or dramatic change in their look. We hope this book has given you the foundation needed to provide these services to your clients, and we wish you the best of luck as you venture into these new areas!

INDEX

NOTES